IMPROVING WITH AGE
WHAT EXERCISE CAN DO FOR YOU

RISTEÁRD MULCAHY

LIB
ERT
IES

CONTENTS

ACKNOWLEDGEMENTS

I am grateful to Ulick O'Connor for the consistent encouragement and advice he gave me during the writing of this *parvum opus*. I wish to thank Aidan O'Hanlon, Emer Shelley, Oliver McCullen, Eamon Ryan TD, Aidan O'Hanrahan of the Central Statistics Office, Jeroem Buis and Michael Aherne of the Dublin Transportation Organisation, Cyril Forbes and Lorcan Walshe for their advice and assistance. I am grateful as always to Michael O'Shea, Maureen Mulvihille and Adrienne Egan of the Irish Heart Foundation, and to Orna Somerville of the UCD Archives for her initiative in helping to arrange publication. Richard and Hugh Mulcahy solved the more arcane aspects of computerology, while my wife, Louise, was a patient observer and a helpful critic. Barbara Mulcahy helped with the typescript, while Seán O'Keeffe and Peter O'Connell were ideal partners in the publication process.

The publishers would like to thank W. H. Freeman & Co., New York, for granting permission to reproduce the figures that appear on pages 113 and 127 and for the material contained in the table on page 115, all of which originally appeared in *Vitality and Ageing: Implications of the Rectangular Curve*, by James F. Fries and Lawrence M. Crapo.

FOREWORD

In the 1950s, when US president Dwight D. Eisenhower was stricken with a coronary heart attack, much attention focused on his subsequent recovery programme. Instead of cutting down on exercise, as had been common practice for those recovering from heart attacks up to then, he was advised by his physician, Dr Paul White, to embrace it vigorously and adopt a regular bicycle-riding programme as well as to continue to play golf. Attention focused on this approach, which now forms the basis for modern treatment of heart disease. In 1966, Risteárd Mulcahy and his colleagues in the Irish Cardiac Society set up the Irish Heart Foundation. Later he was joined by Noel Hickey and Ian Graham in the health-promotion work of the foundation. Ireland had one of the highest rates of death from lung cancer and heart disease in the world.

The Irish Heart Foundation, over the next fifty years, would play a big part in reducing not only heart disease but lung cancer and other illnesses as well. The foundation focused on the destructive effects of cigarette smoking and the dangers of large intakes of saturated fat, such as is found in butter and meat. They also presented to the public a high profile on exercise as a means of reducing blood pressure and cholesterol. As a result of their efforts, there has been a substantial decline in deaths from heart disease in Ireland today. Now, Professor Mulcahy has written an absorbing book which holds one from start to finish and which embodies many of the ideas that underlie the programme of the Irish Heart Foundation.

Risteárd Mulcahy has a perfect answer for anyone who might chide him with the phrase 'Physician heal thyself.' He has only to point to his own excellent physical condition. He tells us that, in his eighty-second year,

9

his interest in exercise has 'increased rather than decreased over the years and has left me with the happy delusion that I am improving with age.'

He had been a fine golfer (playing off a handicap of seven) in his twenties, a member of an excellent University College Dublin rowing eight, and later a committed squash player. But it wasn't until he was in his fifties that he came to recognise the specific benefits of running and, becoming devoted to this form of exercise, went on to run his first marathon at sixty. From then on, no matter where he went, now he brought his running shoes with him. However demanding his professional schedule might be, he would adapt it to his running needs. Today he recalls as his most satisfying run the one 'from Fisherman's Wharf in San Francisco to the Golden Gate Bridge, across to Sausalito and back to San Francisco Park, a distance of nine miles.'

He writes very well indeed of the enhancement of the spirit that ensues from running, and of the communion with nature that the sport provides. His favourite Dublin run was in the early morning from his house near Lansdowne Road along the Sandymount nature park by the sea until he reached the Poolbeg lighthouse at the end of the pier, when he would turn and run back: 'To do this run very early on a fine summer's morning, with the sun rising above Howth Head and without a soul around, was a euphoric experience which transcended my day-to-day life. The gathering warmth, the surrounding seascape and the whiff of the ocean, the far-off Wicklow Mountains in the early-morning mist, the birdsong and the wilderness of the nature park were evocative of our close association with and dependence on nature. The quiet surroundings and the brightness of the distant houses in Irishtown and Sandymount belied the frenetic nature of our urban lives.'

The author descibes the hedonistic feeling and

rush of pleasure that exercise can engender and explains in clinical terms how the brain produces endorphins, which have 'an opium-like effect in reducing pain and provoking feelings of pleasure.' It is heartening to have such fascinating information from a distinguished physician who has himself experienced the chemical metamorphosis he describes.

Perhaps it is because our society is post-colonial that we sometimes find it difficult to take on the responsibilities of commitment necessary for long-term achievement. No society can improve without the creation of insitutions which provide continuity and growth. Risteárd Mulcahy has identified himself with challenges of this kind. It may be an inherited trait, as it was a distinctive element in the career of his father, General Richard Mulcahy, to seek solutions which were likely to have a prolonged and beneficial effect on the body politic. As the first chief of staff of the Irish revolutionary army and as chief of staff and subsequently commander in chief of the Free State army from 1922 to 1924, he had shown a similar vision and an ability to achieve long-term results. In addition, the Mulcahy family and friends have created the magnificent Richard Mulcahy Town Park in Clonmel on land provided by Clonmel County Council. The Romans had a word for this: *pietas.*

Risteárd Mulcahy is the author of books of biography and history as well as having written on the environment and medical matters, and has the fortunate gift of being able to convey to his readers a vigorous personality expressing itself in clear and fluent prose. The present book combines an entertaining personal narrative with first-hand scientific information about methods that can be used to benefit our health, and as well, the writer has tested his conclusions in the forge of his own personal experience. Enjoy it.

Ulick O'Connor

11

AUTHOR'S INTRODUCTION

I ran my first marathon in 1981 during my sixtieth year. Covering just over twenty-six miles through the streets of Dublin was the toughest experience of my life – with the possible exception of a few early rowing ordeals when I was at university. I hit 'the wall' after twenty miles of this first marathon and suffered agonies during the last six miles. It seemed utter madness at the time, but it proved to be a seminal moment in my life. It confirmed for me the truth, which I had first learnt when rowing, that there is no joy without suffering – that the greater the sacrifice the greater the fulfilment.

For this and other reasons, exercise has played a crucial part in my life. It has maintained my mental and physical stamina and has improved my self-image and sense of well-being. My interest in exercise has increased rather than decreased over the years, and at my current age of eighty-one it has left me with the happy delusion that I am improving with age. It has inspired me to be a public advocate of exercise as the road to achieving health and happiness, just as it has inspired me to write this book.

I started writing about my experiences of exercise on my seventy-first birthday, 13 July 1993. After a long interregnum, I completed it after my eighty-first birthday in 2003. I went for a five-mile run on that evening in 1993 after seeing a few patients at my clinic, and before my birthday dinner. It was then that I conceived the idea of writing about exercise and physical fitness and what they have meant to me over the course of my lifetime, with the aim of sharing my personal and professional experiences in relation to health care with a wider audience. The importance of aerobic exercise in maintaining good health and physical fitness in all age groups should receive more attention through public education, schooling and the provision of adequate exercise and sporting facilities. A life of exercise will ensure a healthy and independent old age and will shorten the final and inevitable period of disability.

PART I

THE IMPORTANCE OF EXERCISE

THE BENEFITS OF AEROBIC EXERCISE

'Exercise is the best medicine'
HIPPOCRATES

In evolutionary terms, exercise is a natural part of the human condition. It was a key element in the history of mankind until the beginning of the industrial revolution in the nineteenth century. The very design and extraordinary adaptability of the human frame are consistent with the view that humans are biologically intended to lead active physical lives. The response of muscle strength and mass to training, the considerable reserves of heart, lung and other organ functions, which allow extreme and prolonged aerobic exercise, all bear witness to the part exercise and hard physical work played in the lives of our forebears, in many cases as recently as fifty years. But things have changed dramatically with the coming of industrialisation and more recently with the mass adoption of mechanical methods of transport and physical labour.

In talking about the benefits of exercise on health and longevity, I am largely dealing with leisure exercise. Studies have, however, confirmed that work exercise is also beneficial in reducing mortality from heart attacks and high blood pressure. Sadly, physical exercise at work is now almost a thing of the past, as is evident from increasing levels of obesity among American blue-collar workers and among their equivalents in Ireland. Today the ubiquitous use of the car, the television and the computer has created a sedentary society which is in striking contrast to the active society I knew in my early days. A great deal of heavy work is now carried out by machines, while the workers themselves are in many cases overweight or obese; this was rarely seen in the days preceding the use of machinery. It should be noted, though, that obesity is increasing among all occupational classes and not only among the former labouring classes. This would suggest that, in relation to obesity, non-work lifestyle factors are as important as work-related factors. The phenomenon of mass physical inactivity has occurred in a minute fraction of the millions of years in which there has been human life on earth. This phenomenon has had little effect so far on our bodily design and function but if exercise ceases to be a fundamental part of our lives, it must surely lead to key changes in the human frame and its functions.

In writing about exercise, I define it as aerobic: that is, exercise requiring mobility, increased oxygen consumption and energy output, and increased heart and lung fitness. This is also called isotonic exercise, as opposed to isometric exercise, where the exercise is static and is designed to build up and strengthen muscle rather than lead to cardio-respiratory fitness. Weightlifting and chopping wood are examples of isometric exercise. These are more appropriate for young people who wish to increase their strength and stamina.

Aerobic exercise, if practised regularly, will lead to improved exercise capacity and physical fitness. It is not to be confused with aerobics, which is a static programme designed to improve flexibility and to induce mood changes such as feelings of tranquillity and relaxation. Aerobics requires little increase in oxygen consumption.

There are valuable psychological and mood benefits to be derived from regular exercise – not unlike those associated with transcendental meditation – and quality of life is enhanced in many ways. Regular exercise over time has an important impact on our health and longevity. It is a major factor in the prevention of coronary heart disease, the single greatest killer in Western countries. The effect of exercise on heart disease is based on its beneficial effects in reducing cholesterol, blood pressure and weight, in preventing and controlling diabetes, and in stabilising the inner lining of diseased coronary blood vessels, which, under certain conditions, may become unstable and lead to clot formation and heart attack. Over the long term too, exercise may contribute to increasing the capacity and extent of the coronary blood vessels and thus to enhancing the blood supply to the heart muscle.

There is no doubt that the adoption of a healthy lifestyle by the masses and the consequent improvement in public health can only be achieved through the introduction of an exercise culture into the country. Such a change can only be brought about by means of public education and a greater commitment by the medical profession to health promotion. We are to an increasing extent becoming viewers of elite sports rather than participants in sport at the grass-roots level. Only public policy can provide the stimulus to reverse this trend. The government and sporting and voluntary organisations have a large part to play here.

In recent years, heart specialists have to an increasing extent grasped the value of exercise. In fact, exercise has been a fundamental part of the heart-management programme at St Vincent's Hospital in Dublin since our coronary heart disease research programme commenced in 1961. In atherosclerosis, or disease of the coronary arteries, the arteries supplying the heart muscle with blood become narrowed or blocked by a gruel-like, cholesterol-rich material, and there is a tendency to clotting. Atherosclerosis was long ago found to be less serious in monkeys with high levels of cholesterol that were exercised regularly on a treadmill than in monkeys that also had high cholesterol but were sedentary. It is not surprising therefore that the same results are being replicated in recent large trials in humans. We have known for a long time that aerobic exercise improves quality of life, reduces the risk of cardiovascular disease through control of high blood pressure and high blood cholesterol, and reduces disability in older people. It is only very recently, however, that research has confirmed that exercise contributes independently to increased longevity by virtue of the fact that it produces hormonal and cellular changes which protect the delicate lining of the heart and the blood vessels of the heart and brain.

Regular aerobic exercise is beneficial in preventing colon, breast and prostate cancer, which are among the commonest cancers in Western society. Such exercise may also influence some other less common cancers. Except for lung cancer and other less common tumours, where the main cause is known, the causes of colon, breast and prostate cancer are not known. Almost certainly multiple factors are involved, some of which are recognised. Recent clinical and epidemiological research, however, is pointing more and more to a sedentary life as being a factor in such cancers. This is not well known to the public – nor indeed to many doctors – as yet. Nonetheless, a perusal of the internet will underline the extensive literature confirming the value of exercise as a definite anti-carcinogenic agent (see page 159).

The musculoskeletal system also benefits from regular exercise. The United States Administration on Ageing has stated that 'disuse is the mortal enemy of the human body'. Exercise has a dramatic effect in reducing disability and decrepitude as we approach the end of our lives, thus ensuring greater independence for the old. It is the most effective measure to prevent bone-softening osteoporosis and its consequent complications of injury and invalidism. Like osteoporosis, arthritis of the large joints is commonly associated with ageing but is less common in people who exercise regularly and in a sensible fashion. In addition, recovery from injury and illness is faster in people who are aerobically fit compared to those who are not.

The critical part physical exercise plays in the prevention and treatment of our commonest diseases, and its role in improving quality of life and preventing undesirable mood changes, has to be seen against the background of the gradual reduction of exercise in the daily lives of people in Western society. Work exercise is virtually a thing of the past, and leisure exercise in the form of walking, jogging, running and ball games is mostly confined to young people. Even within the younger age groups, however, for people at school, those in university and in individuals up to their mid-twenties, there is evidence of diminished exercise activity in all Western countries. This is confirmed by information from many agencies here and abroad, and is also reflected by the alarming increase in overweight and obesity in all age groups, most worryingly among children.

The National Health and Lifestyle Survey, conducted by the Irish Ministry of Health and Children, publishes the various indicators of health in the Irish population every four years. The latest quadrennial survey, which was carried out in 2002, and the results of which were published in April 2003, found that there has been a gradual reduction in the proportion of people who smoke and a corresponding reduction in exposure to passive smoking in public places. The prevalence of cigarette smoking among men has been falling for twenty years or more, while there had been an increase among women, at least until recently. This is reflected in the fall in the reporting of lung cancer in men and the increase in such reporting in women. The latest reports from government sources find that 27 percent of men and women are cigarette smokers.

I have little doubt that the government's decision to ban smoking in pubs, hotels, clubs and similar loca-

21

tions will further add to the falling numbers of people who smoke. This recent legislation has caused much anxiety to pub owners and others but I do not believe their fears of losing customers are justified. It is clear from the results of previous legislation, such as the restrictions on smoking during air travel, that smokers do not suffer withdrawal effects when they find themselves in non-smoking areas. They do not feel the urge to smoke while in church or in other non-smoking areas, but feel the immediate need for a cigarette when they find themselves in locations which they associate with smoking. Smoking is a habit which is related to situation and location as well as to a cyclical chemical effect on the body. From the public-health point of view, the government's decision on smoking in public places is an enlightened one.

There has, however, according to the National Health and Lifestyle Survey, been a further reduction in exercise among all age groups and a corresponding increase in obesity. The only age group with some experience of strenuous exercise is men between eighteen and thirty-five years. Men in this age group are more active than women, and those who have second- and third-level education are more active than those with only first-level education.

The Minister for Health and Children said at the launch of the latest quadrennial report:

> With busy, modern lifestyles, people are finding less and less time for physical activity. Inactivity, coupled with poor eating habits, can lead to overweight and obesity, which are not only serious problems in themselves but can lead to further complications, such as diabetes.

The issue of exercise has important political and social implications. Continued improvements in the motor-transport infrastructure, the gradual reduction in exercise facilities in local communities, the inaccessibility of such facilities due to increasing litigation, and the huge commercial pressures on the public to become viewers of top professional sports – rather than participants in these sports – are some of the reasons for the inexorable reduction of leisure exercise in society. This trend will only be aggravated by the building of more national stadia rather than measures being taken to improve facilities in order to encourage exercise at schools and at community level. Actions that should be taken in this area include extending the national cycle-track grid, the implementation of more enlightened town planning aimed at, among other things, an increase in pedestrianised areas, and the developement of an extensive system of pathways and tracks in the mountains, countryside and forests.

We have many areas of new suburban sprawl in our towns and cities where cycle pathways could be routinely built at little extra cost, to provide safe entertainment and aerobic exercise for both children and adults. Yet, despite the fact that such a recommendation was contained in the report of the Lord Mayor's Commission on Cycling in 1995 (see page 159), no policy relating to the building of cycle paths has been adopted by any of our local authorities, nor have many local authorities or private developers built bicycle pathways in our newer suburbs, despite the opportunity to provide such excellent facilities at little extra cost.

It may be no coincidence that the gradual reduction in aerobic exercise among Irish people is occurring in parallel with increasing television viewing, particularly among young people. Robert Putnam's book *Bowling Alone: The Collapse and Revival of American Community* draws attention to the huge adverse changes which have taken place in American society during the last fifty years in terms of social isolation, lack of exercise, obesity, television viewing and dependence on the car for transportation. Sadly, as the latest Department of Health and Children report confirms, we in Ireland – along with our neighbours in Europe and elsewhere – are inexorably following American trends in terms of reduced exercise and increasing weight. Our American cousins claim to have a better standard of living than ours: if this is so, it is only in terms of material possessions and not in terms of quality of life.

The increasing prevalence of obesity in modern Western society is a precursor of the so-called hypokinetic diseases (the diseases common in the sedentary): coronary heart disease, high blood pressure, diabetes, arthritis and some forms of cancer. The increasing incidence of overweight is largely related to the reduced exercise which is a feature of modern life in the West. Obesity has increased from 15 percent of the United States adult population in 1991 to 27 percent in 1999, and now affects more than 10 percent of Americans under seventeen years of age. European and other developed countries are exhibiting the same trends. It is virtually impossible for an obese person to return to and remain at a normal weight without adopting a realistic and sustained aerobic-exercise programme as well as eating healthily. In the current circumstances, the 'battle of the bulge' cannot be won without a huge cultural change in Western society.

During the past year, obesity and its causes and consequences have received much publicity in Ireland, where the incidence of overweight in children and adults is clearly increasing. Some remedies have been suggested to control this trend, including taxing high-calorie food and introducing dieting regimes, but none are likely to succeed as long as we follow the American model and substitute binge eating and fast food for work and leisure exercise. Only a reversal of the current cultural eating habits is likely to succeed. This will require more drastic solutions: we must look at the advertising of high-calorie foods, the quality of school meals, and we need public education to achieve the cultural changes required to reverse current trends.

Unfortunately, we doctors have no easy remedy for obesity, particularly in its more extreme and intractable forms. The latest diet fad seldom survives the initial enthusiasm that surrounds it. Appetite-suppressing drugs are rarely of permanent value in controlling an individual's tendency to overeating, and surgical operations, which are advised only in very severe cases, are not always successful and may do more harm than good. Psychological intervention may help to motivate patients to maintain a changed lifestyle but only if the subject remains under continuous supervision, either with a therapist or within an organisation such as Weight Watchers or Unislim (see page 159).

The recent extension of services by general practitioners and local authorities in Ireland to provide more nutritionists and obesity clinics is a move in the right direction. Several pharmaceutical companies are also providing practical and educational services to prevent and treat obesity. These developments are clearly highlighting the problem and increasing public awareness of the importance of taking personal responsibility for health.

For children, the only effective approach to overweight is to reduce the amount of time they spend watching television and playing video games, and in particular to reduce the amount of food they eat while doing these things. Such programmes are unlikely to succeed, however, unless there is a drastic change within the adult population as well. Today's trend towards obesity in children is simply a reflection of their parents' habits and lifestyles and of a laissez-faire approach to child management.

During my sixty years as a doctor, innumerable weight-reducing diets have been advocated, tried and tested, and sometimes adopted worldwide. Adherence to these diets has rarely persisted beyond the early days of desperation, largely because unnatural food habits are unlikely to be adhered to without difficulties in long-term compliance and because of failure to adopt a more holistic approach to the problem of overweight. Dieting alone is unlikely to achieve a permanent return to a more satisfactory weight level without an increasing expenditure of energy as well as the maintenance of a moderate energy intake. Successful weight loss over the long term is unlikely without the adoption of an adequate programme of aerobic exercise.

It is clear from population studies that physically active people are substantially lighter than those who are sedentary. The first and most practical step in dealing with the obese is to insist that they incorporate an aerobic-exercise programme into their lifestyle. Exercise, combined with sensible eating, with an emphasis on fruit, vegetables and other healthy and low-calorie foods, is the most practical approach to this problem.

It is far from easy at times to find the motivation to take part in an effective exercise programme. In my experience, however, a course of counselling may lead to compliance and to successful weight control. Virtually all the diets I have encountered have been faddist and have failed because they are not consistent with everyday living within the community.

Moreover, a number of community exercise facilities, such as school gyms, are no longer available to the wider public because of a fear of litigation on the part of the owners of the facilities. Ireland needs legal reform to protect *bona fide* sports providers from mischievous and opportunistic litigation.

I am convinced that the only real solution to the problem of obesity will occur when society respects the lean and the active, while looking askance at the fat and inactive, and when public opinion leads government and industry to support more exercise and healthier nutrition. Food labeling, informative advertising, and proper choice should be the rule in our retail outlets, for instance. I believe that the prevalence of the eating disorders bulimia and anorexia nervosa is the product of our current undisciplined eating habits and that a change in society's attitudes, with the development of a more rational approach to eating and exercise, would help to reduce or eliminate these abnormal eating conditions.

Can such cultural changes take place in Ireland while we are bombarded by advertising which urges us to eat more, to eat more often and to eat fast foods high in calories, and while we become more dependent on television for entertainment and on the car for getting around? Without a profound cultural change in attitudes and an equally profound change in the food and advertising industries, it is unlikely that we can reverse current trends.

The USA has led the field in the increasing obesity trends across the Western world – a trend that contimues to the present day. Things are little better in Ireland. In a comprehensive survey by Dublin City University in the East Coast region, 70 percent of adolescent females and 58 percent of adolescent males were found not to take regular exercise. Of the total group, 25 percent were found to be overweight or obese. A SLAN report from University College Galway confirmed that exercise among teenagers and adolescents had fallen between 1998 and 2002; this certainly presages increasing obesity among these groups.

The increasing weight and obesity implications for society were dealt with recently in detail by the international task force of the European Association for the Study of Obesity. They describe this phenomenon as a European epidemic. Fifty percent of the citizens of the

European Union are overweight; of these people, half are obese. We define weight by the Body Mass Index (BMI) - weight in kilogrammes multiplied by height in centimetres squared. Someone with a BMI of between 26 and 30 is overweight, while a person with a BMI greater than 30 is classified as obese. Another method of gauging whether someone is overweight is to measure their maximum waist circumference: greater than thirty-four inches in women and greater than forty inches in men indicates overweight. You can check your BMI by logging on to the VHI website (see page 159).

Due to the recently reported abrupt increase of type 2 diabetes among children in Europe, the task force urges us to listen to the alarm bells about obesity. This is not to mention the increased threat to health among older victims of obesity: high blood pressure, diabetes, heart and gall-bladder disease, cancer of the breast, colon and prostate, and a variety of disabilities including back trouble, arthritis, gout, reduced exercise capacity, sleep apnoea (snoring), hormone disturbances, polycystic ovarian syndrome, impaired fertility and, possibly, reduced libido.

Apart from the calories burnt through the energy expenditure achieved, exercise will help an obese person to overcome the habit of overeating by suppressing an over-demanding appetite. Exercise, and particularly strenuous exercise, helps to control over-eating. Moreover, there is increasing pressure from the European Union and health ministers to encourage the food industry to reduce the calorie content of foods, and on the advertising industry to be more socially responsible.

*

Exercise also offers numerous benefits for pregnant women and their babies. Aerobic exercise contributes to the health of the unborn baby as well as to the mother. Regular symptom-limited walking is strongly encouraged, at least during the first five or six months of pregnancy. Exercise capacity tends to fall gradually from the sixth month of pregnancy, although non-weight-bearing exercise, such as swimming and cycling, can be continued into the later stages without the same fall in capacity. The calisthenic type of exercises which are prescribed by obstetricians and midwives are also to be encouraged later in pregnancy.

Aerobic exercise reduces the level of blood pressure in the pregnant woman and has been reported to be associated with shorter labour. In some reports there has been a lower incidence of Caesarean section among active women compared to sedentary women. Like other people, expectant mothers should of course respond to warning signs of overexertion, such as pain, excessive fatigue, unusual breathlessness and dizziness.

Apart from the physical benefits associated with it, there is some evidence that exercise during pregnancy is associated with enhanced self-esteem and body image as well as with improved appetite and sleep. There is no doubt that women who are aerobically active during pregnancy feel better than those who are sedentary. The benefits of exercise in pregnancy should not surprise us when we recall the history of pregnant women who continued heavy physical work right up to delivery in more primitive and early societies.

The Physiology of Exercise

Exercise requires the expenditure of physical energy. Physical training involves complex physiological changes in the muscles, heart, lungs, blood vessels, and in the blood, which carries oxygen. These changes are aimed at increasing the efficiency of oxygen supply, transport and utilisation, and the production of energy to increase strength, stamina, durability and flexibility. The limiting factor in whole-body exercise is the capacity of the heart to deliver oxygen. Heavy weight training in a young person may increase muscle mass and strength two or three-fold; complete inactivity, as occurs after injury or among astronauts, can lead to muscle wasting of 20 percent or more within a few weeks.

Muscle mass in a sedentary person begins to decrease at about the age of twenty-five. By the age of fifty, it may be reduced by 10 percent, and by the age of eighty, by 50 percent. Regular training such as weightlifting lessens the loss of mass and strength.

Some people are more efficient at sustained exercise while others are more efficient sprinters. This depends on the type of muscle fibre which is dominant in the leg muscles. Extensive research in recent years confirms that there are three types of muscle fibre: a slow one called type 1, a fast one called type 2x and a medium one called type 2A. The average person has an equal amount of the three types in the large muscles of the thigh. Top sprinters have a predominance of the fast type, 2x, while in long-distance runners the slow type, type 1, will dominate.

It is possible that, by means of prolonged training, some changes can be induced in the proportion of these three types. A sample of muscle – a biopsy – can be taken to determine whether you are a sprinter or a long-distance runner, or a mixture of both. Younger people who may wish to take up competitive running or walking might wish to consult a sports specialist to arrange such a biopsy.

With exercise training, muscle mass, and the number and size of blood vessels in the muscle, increases. Muscle becomes more efficient at extracting oxygen from the blood and utilising the energy sources of fat and sugar extracted from the blood. The muscles of the leg in highly trained runners can extract as much as twenty times the volume of oxygen as resting muscle. The increase in oxygen consumption is directly proportional to the degree of training done. An increase in muscle mass is particularly likely to occur in children and younger adults in response to repeated and sustained usage and is specific to the muscles involved. This phenomenon can be seen in the active upper limb of professional tennis players and in the shoulder muscles of lumberjacks (before the advent of the chainsaw). The ability to increase muscle mass decreases as we get older, and eventually, even in an older person who trains regularly, the inevitable slow attrition of ageing leads to a slow loss of muscle mass.

Muscle can reduce in mass by as much as 20 percent in a few weeks when immobilised by concomitant injury, and it may be slow to recover. There is also a beneficial effect on heart muscle among highly trained athletes, leading to an increase in muscle mass and an increase in the bore, or width, of the coronary vessels. The heart, too, becomes more efficient at extracting oxygen and utilising sugar and fat.

Exercise and training bring about complex changes in bone as well as muscle, and strengthen joint cartilage and ligaments. Most important for the elderly, exercise is a powerful antidote to osteoporosis because of the increased bone density created by the effect of stress-

31

loading and weight-bearing. Low levels of exercise lead to a fall in bone density. For instance, some days spent confined to bed will provoke a loss of bone-building calcium from bone and a detectable reduction in bone density, with a consequent loss of strength and a greater risk of fractures.

The increase in bone density is largely confined to weight-bearing exercise; swimming and calisthenics do not confer the same benefit. The benefit also tends to be specific to the structures involved in exercise – the leg bones in walkers and runners, the arm bones in tennis players, and all the major bones in oarsmen.

THE PSYCHOLOGICAL EFFECTS OF EXERCISE

The psychological benefits of physical exercise are at least as important as the physical benefits. The United States National Institute of Mental Health has summarised the effects of exercise on mood and therefore on quality of life. This body has reported that aerobic exercise and physical fitness:

1   contribute positively to mental health and well-being
2   reduce stress emotions such as anxiety states
3   reduce mild to moderate anxiety and depression caused by failure to cope
4   reduce traits such as neuroticism and hypochondria
5   are a useful adjunct to other methods of treating severe depression
6   help to reduce heart rate, stress hormones, neuromuscular tension and other stress indices, and improve sleeping patterns
7   confer benefits extending to all ages and both sexes.

It is not generally realised that children who are inactive are particularly prone to mood changes and adverse psychological effects. This phenomenon may have as much to do with the lack of social adhesion provided by exercise and sport, and consequent social isolation, as the lack of physical exercise per se. People who do not take part in sport also fail to achieve the feeling of fulfilment which is an inherent part of exercise, physical fatigue and competition.

The mechanism in the brain which accounts for the psychological benefits associated with exercise and fitness is not fully understood, but it is likely that a number of chemical changes may be involved. The endorphins are protein substances produced in the brain that have an opium-like effect in reducing pain and provoking feelings of pleasure. The word 'endorphin' is derived from 'endogenous morphine', 'endogenous' meaning 'from within'. This substance is produced by the brain and has a morphine-like effect. The addiction to exercise experienced by the dedicated runner or walker may be similar to an addiction to morphine.

Endorphins are produced in response to certain drugs, intense physical exercise and perhaps sexual activity. Increased endorphin production may be the mechanism whereby pain is relieved through acupuncture and other complementary methods of treatment. This may account for the pleasure enjoyed during aerobic exercise and for the placebo response noted in patients who respond to suggestion, and to the benefit exercise training may have in patients suffering from depression.

We know that some of the monoamine chemicals in the brain are altered by exercise in the same way as they are affected by the psychotropic drugs which are commonly used in the treatment of depression. There is an extensive literature on this subject which supports the value of graduated aerobic exercise and physical fitness in coping with the many mood changes people encounter in modern society.

As regards individual competitive sports, such as tennis and golf, confidence is the key to success; the ingredients of confidence are concentration, being focused, and avoiding all distractions in thought and deed. Of course, practice and training will also contribute to confidence. Forget about both your opponent and the outcome of the match. Instead, think about the shot in hand – not about the last one or the next one but the one you are playing. Your approach should be meditative and tranquil, and not excitable, arrogant, or fearful of failure. Relaxation techniques may be valuable to allay anxiety, reduce tension and provide a sense of detachment.

Confidence is equally important in team sports, where success depends as much on team spirit, loyalty to colleagues, club or country, and harmony among team members as it does on ability and skill. Felicity Heathcote, in her book *Peak Performance*, quotes Chris Pym, the Leinster rugby player: 'When we play as a team, we all do well.' Her book is recommended for those who aspire to perfection in sport (and indeed in other walks of life); it has a good chapter on relaxation techniques.

PART II

A LIFE OF EXERCISE

Early Days

At school, I took no part in active or competitive sport, although there was considerable emphasis there on the two Gaelic games, football and hurling. There was less interest in athletics. Games introduced by the British, and particularly the British army, were strictly forbidden by our teachers, the Christian Brothers. Any pupil in my Irish-speaking school, Coláiste Mhuire in Dublin, who was reported to have been playing rugby or soccer would be severely admonished and banned from the school teams. In fact, my cousins, who attended the school, and perhaps many others, did play soccer and other 'foreign' games, but did so clandestinely and during the evenings or at weekends. At this time, the Gaelic Athletic Association Vigilance Committee was actively rooting out such offenders. Independence had little effect on the social and sporting life of Dublin, however, which in many ways retained the mores of the earlier British regime.

Younger people nowadays are puzzled by the attitude of the GAA at that time. Indeed, it is only in recent times that an easing of these restrictive attitudes has become evident. Virtually the last resistance by the GAA to 'foreign' influence was overcome in 2001, when members of the British forces in the North of Ireland, who had previously been banned from playing Gaelic games, were admitted to the organisation. All that now remains is for the GAA to permit international soccer and rugby to be played in Croke Park, a proposal which is still being debated but may be resolved soon.

During the 1920s and 1930s, many of the more extreme nationalist people in politics and education shared these xenophobic prejudices about British sport. This attitude is generally attributed to the separatist movement which started during the early part of the century. I do not accept this view, however: I would attribute it instead to the divisions created by the Civil War which followed the Treaty settlement with the British in 1922, and to the sustained anti-Treaty republican propaganda, which charged the supporters of the new state, who were committed to working the Treaty, with being pro-British and anti-national in their outlook and policies. I have little doubt that, without this pressure and the bitter divisions of the Civil War, the Free State and the subsequent Republic would have retained more cordial relations with the British and with our Northern brethren, and we would not have concerned ourselves with attempting to eradicate 'foreign games' from the national psyche.

Apart from the desultory exercise derived from cycling, scouting, and a casual participation in tennis and hurling with my siblings in the five-acre military field adjoining my home, I was a sedentary child, almost certainly because I was so small and light for my age. I was a pygmy among giants during my last years in school and my first two years in college. My height during my first year in college, when I was seventeen, was under five feet three inches, and my weight about ninety-four pounds. In my second year, after my eighteenth birthday, I added about nine inches in height and perhaps forty pounds or more in weight, all in the space of about nine months. My retarded growth and development probably had a genetic basis: my mother recalled that her own brothers, all big men, were slow to reach their full development.

Rowing

I joined the boat club on my arrival at University College Dublin in 1939. Weighing just over ninety pounds and measuring five feet three, I was an ideal candidate for the role of cox. I coxed for my first three years at university. It was a difficult role because, although I was nominally in charge of the eight oarsmen, my diminutive size facing such burly and macho types at first induced in me a feeling of inferiority bordering on fear, which belied my theoretical authority. I had been invited to join the boxing club as a flyweight immediately on arrival in the university but the idea of spending my life being punched, or punching others, did not appeal to me.

In 1943, during my fourth year in college, I found a place on the maiden eight, rowing number two on the stroke side. I was probably light for this position, even in a maiden eight, but what I lacked in weight and muscle I made up for in commitment and in my appreciation of the camaraderie and team spirit which is such an important feature of a crew and of a rowing club. After two years' rowing, first on the maiden eight and in the following year on the junior eight, I retired from the sport to study for my final medical examinations.

Competitive rowing must be one of the toughest sports in terms of the effort involved during training and during races. Rowing may be one of the only sports that involves virtually every muscle system to a maximum degree. It is therefore an ideal aerobic form of exercise, but it is also one of the most strenuous forms of such exercise and is not suitable for every age group.

We trained six days a week for most of the rowing season from January to July. All forms of tobacco and alcohol were eschewed during training, and bed by eleven was an inflexible rule. There was a strict code of

41

honour which obliged us to follow these rules. We were also discouraged from associating with the opposite sex. I assumed that the basis for this was the idea that sexual intercourse would have a deleterious effect on our fitness. If this were true – which seemed unlikely even to my naive mind – it was a precept which was not relevant to such callow and immature youths as we were at the time.

It was a three-mile cycle along the Grand Canal to the boat club in Islandbridge, often into the prevailing wind, and sometimes in rain, hail or snow. Ice on the river and snow in the late winter were more common then. On the few occasions when the river was heavily iced, we were unable to launch the boats but could cycle the mile to Chapelizod and back on the river itself. It is now many years since the river was negotiable on a bike – further evidence of the destruction of nature by human society and of the increasing imbalance between nature and man.

We changed in a draughty and unheated pavilion and rowed two or three times up and down the Liffey between the bridge at Chapelizod and the weir at Islandbridge, a distance of just over a mile. Afterwards we threw ourselves into a cold shower before cycling the three miles back to my home in Rathmines. On the river, we were invariably accompanied by a coach, cycling along the towpath, who ensured that nobody dared slack. Our training increased in intensity leading up to a regatta, which was an occasion for a mixture of anticipation and foreboding. As there was room for only two boats abreast on the Liffey at this point, there was invariably more than one heat, and with separate races for fours and eights, some might find themselves with three or more races in an afternoon. Unless each race was easily won, one would be exhausted by the halfway point – with little option but to keep going to the end. It was at least as exhausting as the 'wall' I was later to experience during my first marathon. Submitting myself to such masochism,

I would vow never to get into a boat again. But within a few minutes of recovery, despair would change to the euphoria of fulfilment, even if one failed to win.

During the early summer months we would attend the two great provincial regattas, in Cork and Limerick, with occasional visits to other less prestigious events. Boats were carried by rail on flat wagons and had to be heaved about by the crew. We were of course strictly amateurs at that time and were obliged to pay our own expenses. Sponsorship was unheard of, and remained so for many more years. It was a time of great austerity but none the less enjoyable for that.

Except for the longer 'Head of the River' race on the Liffey, the standard distance of races was about one and a quarter miles, the duration about six to seven minutes. The amount of energy expended was such as required anaerobic as well as aerobic muscle metabolism. In other words, the amount of oxygen absorbed even by the fittest oarsman was insufficient to satisfy his energy requirements. We therefore suffered acute stress during each race if the two crews were equally matched or if we were seeking to overtake our opponents.

To the present-day student, it may have seemed a spartan way of life, but at the time we had no great feelings of suffering or heroism. Physical exercise was a routine part of our lives then, and the bicycle and tram were the only means of transport. I don't think I ever missed a training session, whether as a cox or as an oarsman – at least not without giving adequate notice of my absence. Failure to turn up would have left the other members of the crew in the lurch. Of all sports, rowing is the one where the individual is most completely subsumed into the group.

It was a wonderful training, not only in achieving physical fitness but also in inculcating a spirit of comradeship and loyalty in the group. My time in the boat club, and my earlier experiences in the boy scouts, played a major part in the development of my character and in preparing me for a career in medicine. In those earlier years, I learnt the satisfaction to be derived from physical hardship, and working and serving with others.

Later, in 1960, after I had returned to Dublin from London as a consultant cardiologist, I was to do my first research project on the effect of exercise training on the metabolism and physique of young male oarsmen. I reported in the *Journal of the Irish Medical Association* that a four-month period of intense physical training at senior-eight level had a marked effect on the physique of young men aged between nineteen and twenty-three. A considerable increase in muscle mass was associated with a relative loss of fat, without any great change in body weight. Benefit was also noted in the blood-cholesterol level.

At that time, exercise did not always receive the approval of the medical profession, and strenuous exercise such as rowing and squash was suspected of causing harmful heart enlargement and damage. We could find no evidence of such an effect in our subjects. Later, as we researched the causes of coronary heart disease, we found that, contrary to prevailing medical opinion, graduated aerobic exercise in the form of walking or jogging was beneficial in treating patients with heart problems and that heart disease was more prevalent in people who were sedentary than in those who exercised regularly.

A More Sedentary Life

From 1945 until 1960, I took little exercise apart from playing golf. I had been a member of Milltown Golf Club since 1939 and of Portmarnock Golf Club since 1954. While I was in London – from November 1946 to September 1950 – I continued to take no exercise whatsoever. Apart from golf, my sedentary habits continued after my return to Ireland. I weighed about a hundred and sixty pounds at this time, still light for my height of over five feet eleven inches but not for my slender, ectomorphic build.

'Ectomorph' is one of three medical terms used to describe body configuration. The ectomorphic person is lean and skeletal: the long-distance runner. The endomorph is fat and rotund: the Japanese wrestler. The mesomorph is muscular and stocky: the weightlifter or second-row forward. Most people share two of these three characteristics to varying degrees: for example, a fairly muscular person who has a tendency to be fat, such as a second-row forward, is an endomorphic mesomorph, while I am a mesomorphic ectomorph: more skeletal than muscular but with no tendency to fat.

During my post-rowing, sedentary years, I had begun to put on excess weight around my abdomen, the forerunner of middle-age spread. I was also plagued by a bad back, which left me partly or totally disabled for a few days at a time. I recall one day in the 1950s being admonished by an older colleague and friend on the staff of the hospital where I worked, St Vincent's in Dublin. He deplored my bad posture and slovenly gait, and encouraged me to pay more attention to my health and fitness. This advice came from a man who was overweight himself and, apart from playing golf in Portmarnock once a week, took no exercise. This was a time when middle-

45

class males in Ireland, after the usual emphasis on sport and competition in school and university, retired to a sedentary existence for the rest of their lives. They often comforted themselves by invoking a prejudice against exercise, except possibly leisurely golf.

This prejudice about the adverse effects of exercise, which was so prevalent among doctors in the mid-twentieth century and much later, was only one of many fashions which were a feature of medical practice before the advent of proper scientific trials. In fact, the advice to heart patients to take prolonged periods of rest and to avoid all further work and vigorous leisure exercise was about the worst they could have received. Scientific trials were virtually non-existent before World War II and most medical practice at the time was based on the unsubstantiated views and dogma of poorly informed and scientifically untrained experts. Recent research based on studies of populations by epidemiologists leaves no doubt that exercise is of huge importance in the prevention and treatment heart disease, a view which has only recently been widely accepted.

My friend's intervention made no impression on me. Clearly at that time I had no interest in my physical health, nor had I any pride in my bodily integrity. I certainly had no commitment to the physical and mental disciplines required to maintain a state of physical fitness. Golf remained my only form of outdoor activity – and the nineteenth hole proved at times to be a par six! My poor physical state continued for a few more years until the winter of 1960–61. I was the quintessential couch potato.

Since 1961, physical exercise and physical fitness have added an important dimension to the quality of my life, not only in augmenting my pride in my physical health and function but also in improving my mental and physical stamina, and my ability to cope with stress. Exercise has made a major contribution to improving my self-confidence. I think that it is difficult to suffer from boredom, with its associated adverse lifestyle habits, if one uses one's physical and mental faculties to the full.

Vigorous physical exercise may have helped me to cope with periods of chronic frustrated sexuality. Exercise and physical fitness stimulate an increased consciousness and a pride in one's body and its functioning, and these feelings may have a sensuous connotation. I found that running and squash, and the fitness I derived from playing them, had a rather paradoxical effect on my sexuality in that such exercise had a sublimating effect at those times in my life when I was sexually frustrated, while it added greatly to my interest and enjoyment of sex when I had a satisfactory relationship with my partner.

SQUASH

In January 1961 there were several heavy falls of snow, and for six weeks, until the end of February, the country was snowbound. Walls of solidified snow as high as five feet lined the streets of Dublin, and all outdoor sports, including golf, were cancelled. A close friend, colleague and golf partner of mine induced me to play a game of squash in the Fitzwilliam Club as a substitute for golf. I did so reluctantly because, when I had attempted to play squash after my return from England in 1950, my efforts had been rewarded with an acute attack of lumbago, as back pain was then described.

On this occasion I played without mishap. We had several games over the following weeks and I soon became addicted to the sport. I was stimulated by the competitive nature of squash, the fact that I did not make the errors which were inherent in my boyhood tennis, and the pleasant social life associated with squash at the Fitzwilliam Club. Moreover, squash was less time-consuming than golf – an important consideration, as I was becoming busier professionally. I found the strenuous exercise squash entailed had the same fulfilling, if somewhat masochistic, quality as the exercise which I had once enjoyed as an oarsman.

With my introduction to squash began a decline in my interest in golf, so that by 1968 I deserted the golf course, with the exception of playing in the Captain's Prize in Milltown every year. Although I had a handicap of seven, I did not return to the game until I retired from St Vincent's in 1988.

Squash added a new dimension to my life. I was increasingly busy with the responsibility of establishing a heart centre and a coronary-care unit in the hospital, as well as, coincidentally, encountering problems in my personal and domestic life. I played squash as often as four or five times a week. At that time, handicaps were in vogue, and I managed to reduce mine to the respectable level of one hand. I became physically fit for the first time since my rowing days. I lost weight and all signs of middle-age spread disappeared. I gradually became conscious of the rhythms, functions and integrity of my body. The physical effort involved in playing squash was not only satisfying from the sensuous aspect: the psychological benefits were immense as well. A hard day's work was made more enjoyable by the anticipation of a game of squash in the evening. The stresses of my professional and personal lives were easier to bear, and my mental as well as my physical stamina improved.

My active squash career lasted from 1961 until the autumn of 1972, when I had reached my fifty-first year. By this time, some of my squash friends had become interested in running, and I was struck by the fact that, as their interest in running increased, their commitment to squash diminished. In the autumn of 1972, I played a game of five sets with a friend and frequent opponent of about the same standard as myself. This proved to be a marathon, with each of the five sets going to a tie-break. We were a highly competitive pair. I cannot remember who won the final game, but I left the court exhausted – although, as usual, mentally exhilarated. This game marked the end of my squash career.

We in the Fitzwilliam Club were among the first generation of Irish people to continue playing squash beyond the age of thirty. I was satisfied that there was no reason that one should not continue to play into middle age. Indeed, some of my squash friends continued to play into their seventies without mishap, but I had doubts about the demands imposed on my body by the sport. I therefore decided that I should take up some gentler exercise with a training effect, such as jogging or running.

49

RUNNING AND JOGGING

Walking, jogging and running have the great advantage that they can be enjoyed at any time, almost anywhere, and at one's own pace. You are not depending on other people for you exercise, and there need be no element of competition. Moreover, an individual of any age can enjoy such exercise as long as it is appropriate in terms of the person's age and ability. For most people who are interested in keeping fit, walking, jogging and running come close to achieving the most satisfactory whole-body effect. Such exercise requires little expenditure on clothes, equipment and subscriptions to clubs or health centres, except for the purchase of a good pair of walking or running shoes – which, with care, will last for several years. Walking can often be combined with work and other useful pursuits. With adequate practice and a sensible programme, all those who persist with a walking or running programme can become addicted to these pursuits. Walking and running are benign addictions which tend to discourage the more harmful ones which afflict people in our society.

*

As I came to the end of my squash career, I had been practising some graduated walking along the lines advocated by Ken Cooper in his book *Aerobics*. Cooper was the great Texan guru of exercise: it was he who was most responsible for the emerging popularity of jogging and running in the 1950s and 1960s. I was therefore not entirely a novice when I made the decision to take up running as a regular form of exercise. Nonetheless, I found sustained running very difficult at the beginning. On several occasions I was obliged to discontinue because of the impression that I was physically unsuited to such activity. I subsequently learned that many people who attempt to take up running are discouraged because of the same belief – a belief engendered by distressed breathing, muscle pains and the physical discomfort of taking on too much before one has developed a training effect. The important ingredient in the training process at this stage is to start slowly and to avoid pushing oneself until one feels the comfort and rhythm of having acquired one's second wind.

When I write about running, I include the slower activity of jogging. There is no clear dividing line between these two forms of aerobic exercise; in fact, physiologically they are the same. The difference is that the jogger travels at five to seven miles an hour; faster than seven miles an hour can be described as running; racing implies a competitive element.

For the first year or so, I had these stop-start experiences, but by 1973 I was sufficiently well trained to run three or four miles without any great discomfort or anxiety. I had learned to achieve fitness by graduated exercise, by walking a hundred steps followed by jogging fifty, and by increasing the proportion of jogging to walking over a few months until I could comfortably jog a few miles without discomfort. I then increased the intensity of running and could, with regular practice, run longer distances. It took me about a year to achieve the degree of fitness required to run comfortably without distress.

By this time, running had become a very important part of my life: like squash, it added a new dimension in physical and psychological terms to my quality of life. By the late 1970s, I was running five to seven miles three or four times a week and had come into contact with the running fraternity at mini-marathons and other events. I was careful to keep to a threshold of activity within which I would experience no more than a slight degree of breathlessness. I had become an addict and suffered withdrawal effects if I did not run for two or three days consecutively.

Running became important to me as a source of relaxation and escape from the stresses and tensions of a busy professional life. It provided a positive feeling of well-being and freedom from my old back trouble. Running also offered a degree of mental and physical stamina which allowed me to work for long periods without fatigue. Moreover, it enhanced my self-confidence and self-esteem. It has been said that the beneficial effects of running are derived from the ultimate union of mind and body.

I might feel an occasional and transient muscular soreness after a long run, but the fatigue I experienced was physical only. Moreover, the physical fatigue resulting from sustained exercise is fulfilling, unlike the fatigue so commonly described in those who are sedentary, where tiredness is stress related or associated with boredom, and is in essence a form of depression. The pleasures of free and untrammeled movement, the joys of physical fitness and physical well-being bordering on the sensuous, and the stamina to face the daily problems and frustrations of life are all experienced by the dedicated runner. Exercise, particularly of a strenuous nature, is in fact an antidote to depression – albeit, unfortunately, little used by psychiatrists who treat this distressing condition.

Running has a certain spiritual connotation: it offers a means of contemplation and an opportunity for knowing oneself. It brought me closer to nature and the elements, and an appreciation of the essential part the natural world plays in our lives, in terms of both our well-being and survival. It was at this stage in my life that I first became involved in the environmental movement. I found myself alienated from modern life, where the desires for amassing money and material possessions, and an indifference to waste, are the dominant characteristics of all social classes.

I was brought up a Roman Catholic in the conservative culture of the early twentieth century. I soon lost all faith in the dogmas and historical rationale of the Church and in the Christian conception of God. I became an agnostic in the sense that I know that there exists a force which created the world, but I am also aware that neither I nor anyone else is likely to identify that force. My religion became closest to that of the Stoics of Greek and Roman times. Theirs was a spiritual movement that was based on virtue and later became the basis for Christian morality. A fundamental part of my faith was an obligation to do all in my power to protect the natural world and our obligations to future generations.

I believe that there is a certain holiness in this communion with nature. Living near the rugby football stadium at Lansdowne Road, my greatest joy was to run along the nearby strand and the adjoining nature park leading to the mile-long South Wall causeway and its red lighthouse far out in Dublin Bay. To do this run very early on a fine summer's morning, with the sun rising above Howth Head and without a soul around, was a euphoric experience which transcended my day-to-day life. The gathering warmth, the surrounding seascape and the whiff of the ocean, the far-off Wicklow Mountains in the early morning mist, the birdsong and the wilderness of the nature park were evocative of our close association with and dependence on nature. The quiet surroundings and the brightness of the distant houses in Irishtown and Sandymount belied the frenetic nature of our urban lives.

At least in Dublin we can give thanks for such splendid areas as Sandymount and Portmarnock, where peace and isolation can be assured within a stone's throw of the tumult of the city. Running alone through the nature park at Sandymount or through the stippled sunshine of the Marlay Park woodlands, I could feel the spirit of nature seeping into me – a communion akin to being in love and being loved

The joys of the surroundings were enhanced by the steady rhythm of my limbs, and the feeling of vibrant muscle and well-being, all ending in a satisfying degree of physical fatigue bordering on the sensuous. I am fortunate to have known such health and freedom. I had learnt a new pride in the integrity of my body and a conscious desire to protect it from self-induced harm or accident. I have always been moved by the beauty and perfection of a runner, male or female, with a well-built body and a running style which conveyed the rhythm and smooth mobility of the healthy human frame. Of course I yearn for the halcyon days when I ran myself but there is considerable consolation in my memories of running and in the more modest exercise and the continued good health I still enjoy.

Another great advantage enjoyed by the dedicated runner is social contact with other runners. It is an egalitarian sport including all classes, ages and races, and both genders. Moreover, for those who are seeking more than simple companionship, there are ample opportunities for more intimate friendships with people who share other interests as well as exercise and physical fitness.

There is no doubt that the motivation to start a long-term exercise programme such as walking, jogging or running is not easy to acquire. When I am supervising exercise tests at my clinic, I always discuss the patient's exercise history with them. The conversation generally goes along the following lines. I ask: 'Do you take much exercise?' They will answer: 'Not as much as I should.' I then ask: 'Well, do you walk as far as the car?' They will laugh and admit that this is about the limit of their exertions. They generally explain that it is a problem of time or circumstances, but this is very rarely a valid excuse. It is really a matter of priorities; when faced with this assertion, most patients will readily – and sheepishly – agree. You can run or walk in the morning or late in the evening before the pubs close, when the streets are quiet. Television hours can be reduced, and the weekends must provide time for exercise – except, perhaps, for the worst type of workaholic (who anyhow requires counseling about his or her whole philosophy of living).

My running was done from my tennis and squash club, the Fitzwilliam Club, or from my home. In the first few months after I had taken up this pursuit, I felt embarrassed running through the streets and being recognised by the odd passer-by. I tended therefore to wear an old pair of pants and a sweater rather than running gear, and I would slow to a walk or stop and look into a garden or shop window if I encountered a bus queue or passing pedestrians. I soon got over such sensitivities, however, and my inhibitions were eventually resolved completely: I became unaware of passers-by, and I had no inhibitions in running through familiar territory sparsely clad in shorts and a singlet.

In the 1970s and 1980s, I travelled abroad about ten or twelve times a year as part of my medical research activities or as a representative of the Irish medical profession on European committees to implement the mutual recognition of medical training and degrees in the six EEC countries. I found running a boon during my travels. I would set out from the hotel in the early morning before meetings commenced or after the meetings had finished. I might otherwise be tempted to find myself in the bar more often than was good for me. Running in strange cities abroad was a wonderful experience. I have a good sense of direction and could do a five-mile run anywhere without fear of being lost. This was an excellent antidote to the boredom of travel and allowed me to see many places which I would not have seen had I been cooped up for the length of my stay in the conference hotel. Quite frequently, colleagues, both male and female, had a similar interest in running, and this added another enjoyable and intimate companionship that was seldom so easily found in the conference room.

I have a large Mercator-projection map hanging in my study with coloured pins marking every place I have run in the world, from Tromso in the Arctic to Manila in the Philippines, from Boston in the United States to Wellington in New Zealand, and from Moscow in Russia to San Diego in California. I have run in Hyde Park, Kensington Gardens and Regents Park in London, the Bois de Boulogne and the Bois de Vincennes in Paris, Central Park in New York and the great Chapultepec Park in the centre of Mexico City – and felt breathless at the latter's elevation of nearly two thousand metres. My most uplifting run was from Fisherman's Wharf in San Francisco to the Golden Gate Bridge, across to Sausalito and back to San Francisco Park, a distance of nine miles, to be met by and receive the hospitality of an old colleague, Colman Ryan, who is a cardiologist in that great city. He had spent a year as my registrar during his training at St Vincent's Hospital in Dublin.

I always faced oncoming traffic when running. This is doubly important when abroad, as it is easy to forget that traffic keeps to the right in many other countries. I tried to remember that runners are injured or die on the road more often from car accidents than from any other cause, and that such events are more likely to occur at night. In one American study, half of the fifty runners reported killed were running at night. The use of reflective clothing at dusk and at night is therefore crucial. I kept my eye on the near wing of all vehicles until they had safely passed me. I also used to carry a short, stout stick in case of encountering unfriendly dogs; I slowed to a walk in their presence, as they are less likely to be excited by the familiar walker than by the less familiar jogger or runner.

We must also not forget the opportunities for running when travelling around Ireland and Britain. The quiet roads and hill tracks of Wicklow, the towpaths along our canals, the many beautiful and tranquil places in the west of Ireland, and the widespread system of pathways and walking routes in most parts of Britain provide endless opportunities for walkers and runners.

I recall a stay in a splendid hotel in Anacapri at the peak of the Italian island of Capri, where I was attending a seminar in honour of Ancel Keys, an American physiologist and one of the great pioneers of research into the causes of heart disease. Every evening after the afternoon session, a friend of mine from Norway and another from Denmark would join me in running the five kilometres from the hotel downhill to the Blue Lagoon. We divested ourselves of our clothes – we wore swimming trunks under our shorts – dived into the sea from the rocks and swam into the Blue Lagoon through its narrow entrance, despite the protests of the boatmen who wished to solicit our patronage. I had never realised that blue could be so blue. The swim was followed by a glass of beer in the adjoining bar; then, in the cool of the evening, we ran up the five steep kilometres to our hotel and to dinner. Such moments added great enjoyment, bordering on euphoria, and a sense of fulfilment to my many trips abroad.

One day I was running along the Moscow River when I met two other runners who were American; otherwise during my two visits to that city I met no runners. In questioning one of my Russian hosts later, I asked why the Muscovites did not run. He replied with great authority that it had been fashionable in Russia but that they soon ascertained that running was dangerous and was best avoided! He may have been right, for I never encountered such hard concrete as that along the Moscow River!

These were still the days of communism: I found some of my Russian colleagues to be very dismissive of Western – or rather, American – culture.

Moscow was a grey city, with many wide boulevards and some large, dismal apartment blocks. The hotel I stayed in during my first visit, the Rossi, was newly built. It was a huge block with 1,500 bedrooms, run like an army camp, with a formidable female commissar in charge of each floor. She was called a 'babushka', the Russian for 'grandmother'. Residents were obliged to report to this woman on arriving and leaving one's room. Moscow had some merit, however. It had the Kremlin, with its vast museum, a few beautiful churches, with their icons, their ornate exteriors and bulbous onion-shaped domes so evocative of the East, and the Pushkin Gallery, with its magnificent Impressionist paintings.

Moscow also had the monumental GUM store close to the Kremlin. This shop had an extraordinary paucity of consumer goods and was grossly inefficient and bureaucratic. Overall, the Russian shops stood in striking contrast to the wasteful and acquisitive society we have at home. At home we seek out everything we want – or think we want, but do not need. Clearly, the Russians at that time of austerity were lucky to find what they needed. I doubt if they were less happy than we were – nor were we in Ireland less happy during the period of strict austerity between 1940 and 1950 compared to during our present-day culture of excess and waste.

As official foreign visitors representing the World Health Organisation, each of us was provided with a young student as a guide during our stay. Their enthusiasm for the job was apparent; their abiding ambition was to learn English and to travel to the West. I had an attractive girl who was attending university and was very attentive, but she drew the line at joining me for a run along the Moscow River!

Although the Muscovites did not run, they certainly walked. The footpaths were crowded with pedestrians, the men uniformly clad in long black coats and slouch hats. I had an eerie feeling because, unlike the undisciplined crowds in the streets of Dublin and London, the pedestrians in Moscow tended to keep to the left, just as our cars do at home. The dark and sober clothing of the walkers, and the aspect of regimentation, were more evocative of a solemn procession than a crowd.

By contrast, East Berlin, with its wall still intact, which I visited on my way home, appeared to have no merit. I stayed at a large, impersonal hotel, which was modern-American in style but more banana-republic in function and facilities. East Berlin was another concrete desert, newly built, with vast box-like apartment blocks lining wide boulevards, and little traffic. The width of the streets made a mockery of the Irish myth that O'Connell Street is one of the widest in the world. The shops were empty of consumer goods, apart from one shop window which was full of motor tyres! My one compensation was my daily five-kilometre run from the hotel to Checkpoint Charlie and back. Imagine my surprise when, on my first arrival at the checkpoint, I found a small, inconspicuous door in the great wall guarded by a single soldier carrying a rifle. No tanks, no machine-guns, no barbed wire and none of the outdoor furniture one might expect to service a battalion of men dedicated to controlling a discontented citizenry.

I must, however, acknowledge the kindness of my colleagues in East Berlin. Although they looked askance at my addiction to running, they provided me with the warmest hospitality under difficult circumstances.

*

I ran my first marathon in Dublin in October 1981. Training for it was arduous and time-consuming, involving four or five hours' running every week, and runs of up to twenty miles in the Phoenix Park on Sundays for a few months before the event. Despite this programme, my preparation proved insufficient. On the day of the marathon, I ran in reasonable comfort until I reached the twenty-mile mark. I then hit the dreaded 'wall'. My limbs turned to lead, my body appeared to be enclosed in plaster of Paris, and every movement required a supreme effort. The experience brought back memories of my rowing days, when I became exhausted before each race had ended. In the case of running, however, the state of exhaustion and physical pain was considerably more prolonged. It convinced me that such extreme exertion performed for any other reason than to escape from a lion was an act of pure folly.

The 'wall' must be the worst form of masochism ever devised. I recall a medical colleague and previously distinguished Irish international rugby full-back, at Merrion Square a mile before the finish. His face was wreathed in a broad smile as he shouted encouragement at me. I had a brief compulsion to smash his face in, which I interpreted afterwards as a feeling of resentment towards the whole of society and not particularly towards my friend! After an interminable nightmare, I reached St Stephen's Green; within two hundred yards of the finish, I collapsed. I lay prostrate on the street – but was acutely aware of the shouts of encouragement mixed with what seemed to me howls of derision from the multitude witnessing the end of the race. The crowd provoked me to half-crawl and half-walk to the finishing line, where I had to be helped through the tunnel and handed into the care of my sons, Richard and David, and other family members. Due to impending hypothermia, I was wrapped in blankets, transferred to the back seat of my son's car and brought home, where I was plied with hot whiskey. Congratulations were tempered with severe admonitions that, now that I had proved myself – and was at the beginning of my seventh decade – it was time for me to grow up! I should give up running and pursue more sedentary interests consistent with my age!

The hot whiskey was welcome and agreeable but did little to relieve the pains in my legs and recurring, severe cramps. Eventually, after I had been helped to bed, I took two Veganins for my leg pains, two tablets of quinine sulphate to relieve the cramps – an excellent antidote – and two tablets of Valium to allow me to sleep. With this cocktail of drugs, I fell into a deep sleep and remained out for the count for twelve hours. Through a supreme effort of will-power – and the same stubbornness which had seen me finish the marathon – I went into the hospital and did rounds the next morning, trying to conceal my limp and avoid wincing with the pain in my calf muscles and thighs.

I ran my first marathon in four hours and twenty-five minutes. I ran my second in Dublin in 1982 in four hours and twenty minutes. On the second occasion, I did not hit the 'wall' and I was able to fend for myself after I had completed the race. In 1983, I ran my third and last marathon in Belfast. Before doing so, I spent two weeks on vacation in my brother Seán's cottage in Clara, County Wicklow. I ran every day and on several occasions did a run of more than twenty miles. This included some tough running up Trooperstown Hill and along the many roads and slopes between Rathdrum, Glenealy and Clara. I enjoyed the contemplative ambience of my surroundings, the tranquillity and beauty of the Avonmore river valley, and the surrounding hills and woodlands.

The hill-running must have been of considerable benefit, because I completed the Belfast marathon in three hours and fifty minutes, a reduction of thirty minutes compared to my previous best. This marathon was positively enjoyable, even during the race, although I was worried about the prospect of hypothermia while running towards Ormeau Park along the Lagan into a cold north-east wind. Nevertheless, I finished fresh and in good form, and I was able to stand about at the finish with a pint of Guinness in one hand and a sandwich in the other.

My contrasting experiences of running marathons were a stark reminder of the importance and value of proper training. This applies to all aerobic exercise, including walking. It is remarkable how the human body adapts to training at all ages, as long as the training programme is properly graduated. Some of my more obsessive running friends were doing marathon runs of fifty miles at this time.

I attended the Belfast marathon with Barton Kilcoyne, another aficionado of running and one who was influential in my developing an addiction to the sport. He hired a comfortable car and a driver in Dublin; after a successful run in Belfast, we returned to a friend's house to celebrate. This friend, Michael Scott, a cardiologist in the Belfast City Hospital, also ran in the marathon and beat me by only a minute or two. We drank quantities of champagne, disported ourselves like schoolboys, full of pride in our success, and eventually about midnight collapsed into the back seat of our BMW in a delicious state of fatigue and euphoria, and returned to Dublin.

That was my last marathon and my personal best in terms of time. I must have come to my senses or matured in some way after this event. The Belfast marathon was particularly enjoyable and fulfilling because of my friendship with Barton and Michael, and due to the great appreciation shown by the northerners as a result of our participation in their event. Whatever

about their political affiliations, they have the same outlook on life, the same hedonistic capacity to enjoy themselves – and, I suspect, the same genes as ourselves in the
south.

There was one amusing incident which occurred
in Sandy Row, about three miles from the start. As I was
getting into a good rhythm, I heard faintly in front of me
a clop-clop-clopping sound. On reaching its source, I
found a medical colleague from Dublin who was noted
for his commitment to running and who had already
completed at least a hundred marathons, both in Ireland
and abroad. He was dedicated to 'junk' running and
masochism. He had apparently left Dublin early that
Bank Holiday morning and forgotten his running shoes.
No shops were open and he was unable to get shoes on
his way to Belfast. He was therefore obliged to run in his
brown, leather-soled shoes – the source of the clopping
sound.

I spent a few moments running beside him and
commiserating with him. I then excused myself so that I
could return to my former faster pace; the clopping sound
soon receded. I had forgotten about my colleague and his
predicament until I was within a mile or two of the finish.
Again I could hear the distant clopping, becoming ever
louder, until I was finally passed by him a few hundred
yards before the finish! He had run the 26.2 miles in his
ordinary footwear in a fraction less than three hours and
fifty minutes, an achievement I did not think was possible. It would be interesting to learn of his subsequent
health, and particularly the state of his musculoskeletal
system, when he finally hangs up his running boots!

During my active years as a hospital doctor in
Dublin, I was increasingly involved in preventive medicine and health promotion but I earned my living as a
physician and clinical cardiologist. By this I mean that I
spent my time in hospital with patients taking their his-

tories, examining them and making decisions with them and their families about the management of their various conditions. Much of my time was spent dealing with emergency heart attacks. Unlike many latter-day cardiologists, I was not involved in doing tests and spending my time in a laboratory.

My regular work at St Vincent's Hospital entailed ward rounds every Monday, Wednesday and Friday morning. On Wednesday, I would spend three hours or more seeing patients in the coronary-care ward and visiting patients in the other hospital wards at the request of, and in consultation with, colleagues. On each of these rounds, and particularly on Wednesdays, I was accompanied by a 'comet's tail' of young resident doctors, nurses, students and the odd visitor from outside my team or occasionally from abroad. I always sat beside each patient when discussing their symptoms and complaints or listening to the report of the young resident doctor who was responsible for the patient's day-to-day medical care. This procedure took place before an examination of the patient was carried out. All the others in the group were obliged to stand during the rounds, and on rare occasions one of the members of the attending group fainted due to prolonged standing. Fortunately, the resuscitation team attached to our service never needed to intervene.

At the time I was running marathons during the early 1980s, I was still working in the hospital. Naturally, I was much fitter than many of my younger colleagues. After rounds in the coronary-care unit, which was on the ground floor of the hospital, I would visit the general wards to consult with colleagues about their patients. The semi-private ward, St Michael's, was on the top floor. I usually had a patient or two there and would commence my peripatetic consultations by running up the four flights of stairs to St Michael's Ward. I became an expert at concealing my breathlessness when I reached the top of the four flights – and I had a brief moment to recover before the others arrived, invariably distressed and sometimes a little embarrassed by their failure to keep up with somebody twice their age. It was a rare moment of one-upmanship.

I continued running and remained captivated by the sport until I was obliged to stop in 1994 because of arthritis of the left hip. I was in my seventy-third year. Although I ran no more full marathons after 1984, I did a number of half-marathons (twenty-one kilometres) and mini-marathons (ten kilometres). In my early years I ran with other people, but later I almost always ran alone. This allowed me to stay at my own comfortable pace of about 7.3 miles per hour without impeding younger companions. In my last years involved with the sport, I ran about three times a week, doing four to six miles each time. Even less would have been sufficient to maintain a training effect and prevent any withdrawal effects.

After one prolonged non-running period as a result of a soft-tissue injury, I found the training effect I had acquired persisted to some degree. The same is evident with other forms of aerobic exercise. Recovery of fitness can be achieved even after a period as long as six months, but retraining will always be necessary and will need to be graduated in intensity. The loss of cardiovascular fitness may be delayed, however, by adopting other types of exercise programmes. This is why I have always adopted an eclectic approach to exercise.

Now that I have finished with running, I plan each week's exercise by walking two to four miles three times a week. I also play eighteen holes of golf twice a week, cycle maybe once or twice, and take one day off without aerobic activity but with my regular ten minutes of calisthenics in the morning.

Various tests of fitness show that an active man of sixty years has the same heart, lung and musculoskeletal function, and the same mobility and stamina, as the sedentary man of forty years. The same applies to women. In fact, the deterioration in function of all our organs right up to old age is extremely slow if these organs are properly used. This applies particularly to the musculoskeletal and cardiovascular systems. A few people comment on my agility, and the youthfulness of my gait and figure, even though I am now in my eighty-second year. This can only be due to the regular and strenuous aerobic activity which I have done during the last forty years.

All is not lost for the sedentary person, however, irrespective of their age. The sedentary man or woman of forty, with the physical capacity of an active person of sixty, can later, with appropriate training, become the sixty-year-old with a functional capacity perhaps closer to a person of forty years. It is never too late to start.

A satisfactory degree of fitness can be achieved by quite moderate exercise, through either brisk walking or jogging at five or six miles an hour. Those who run long distances regularly may have the fulfilment of doing a marathon or half-marathon but, from the point of of view of fitness compatible with optimum health and well-being, such 'junk mileage' is not necessary.

*

Around 1980, I suffered an injury to my right knee and was unable to run for about six months. The diagnosis was never clearly established, but it appeared to be a soft-tissue injury which was probably extra-articular, that is, outside the joint cavity. Although the specialists whom I consulted advised me to give up running, after six months' rest I made a full recovery and returned gradually to my former activities; this trouble has never recurred.

During my period of enforced inactivity, I maintained regular calisthenic exercises at home. These at least helped to maintain my flexibility and sense of physical coherence. I was surprised, when I resumed running, how quickly I recovered my fitness and capacity for exercise; I was fairly tentative during the early days of my return to exercise, however.

This event was a reminder that soft-tissue sports-related injuries are not uncommon and that the exact cause of such injuries can be difficult to identify. X-rays may be unhelpful, although recent developments in radiology, such as magnetic resonance imaging (MRI) and ultrasonography, are making a huge contribution to more exact diagnosis. Generally, unless the diagnosis is clear and there is some other treatment which may be effective, any problem associated with pain is best treated by rest. As in my case, X-ray evidence of arthritis of the knee, which caused one doctor to advise me to stop running, did not accurately predict the long-term, normal functioning of the joint.

A few years later, I suffered from pain in my right lower back or lumbar region. This pain was episodic and continued for almost a year; it was not sufficiently disabling to cause me to stop running. In fact, the condition was relieved rather than aggravated by running. It never presented with the more serious manifestations of disc trouble. Nevertheless, it was a source of concern to me, and I feared that running might have a long-term adverse effect on the condition.

I consulted several experts but no definitive diagnosis was arrived at until I paid a visit to a well-known sports-injury specialist in Washington, DC. After carrying out a thorough examination of my entire spinal system, he confidently advised me that my trouble was caused by arthritis of an apophyseal joint in the lumbar region, and that I had nothing to be concerned about and should continue running. The apophyseal joints are found between the cantilevered, bony projections which link contiguous vertebral bodies and which are important in allowing the vertebral column to bend and rotate, and yet remain stable. The specialist advised me to stop the various spinal exercises I had been doing. I still get mild apophyseal discomfort, particularly in my neck, but, unlike disc trouble, it causes me little disability. It is the price I pay for the privilege of being alive and still physically active as my musculoskeletal system ages.

This complaint, and the experiences of other people I have met over the years, has made me cautious about calisthenic exercises involving marked rotation and bending of the spinal column. Back and neck exercises of this sort should be confined to movements within comfortable limits.

Shortly after my seventy-first birthday in 1993, I noticed that a discomfort in the region of my left hip, which appeared at the end of a golf round or after running a few miles, and which had started insidiously, was becoming more easily induced and more intense. I suspected that I had early arthritis of the hip joint. The X-ray of the pelvic area and the hips was normal, however, apart from some osteoarthritic changes in my lumbar spine – not unexpected in one of my age. My rheumatologist found slight limitation of movement of the left hip and could not rule out early hip arthritis. In view of the normal X-ray and the relatively mild and inconstant symptoms, however, he felt that no urgent action was required. Various soft-tissue-injury conditions, such as fascio-iliitis, were mentioned by others. These suggestions led to the suspicion that the trouble was caused by my new golf swing.

Since the earlier part of the year, I had been attempting to initiate my golf downswing by bringing the left side of my body through early and forcefully in order to increase the length and accuracy of my tee shots. This action might easily put an excessive strain on the ilio-femoral fascia or on the lateral ligament of the left hip joint in a right handed-person, particularly one of my age. After three months' rest from running, there was a complete resolution of symptoms. During this time, I played less golf but continued some simple calisthenics, with about thirty minutes' tough cycling on my ergometer twice or three times weekly.

The symptoms reappeared soon after I resumed walking and running, however. Over the next few months, the pain and discomfort increased rapidly in intensity, particularly in bed at night. The limited movement of the hip joint had become more evident, and the diagnosis, despite a relatively normal X-ray, was no longer in doubt – nor was the prospect of surgery. If I was to remain completely sedentary, the progress of my symptoms would certainly have been slower, and indeed the condition might have remained almost asymptomatic for an indefinite period. I decided, however, that a hip replacement rather than an enforced sedentary existence was the lesser of two evils. This was the correct decision. Before surgery, I continued some limited walking, and regular sessions on the bicycle ergometer. I retained some of my previous fitness, at least as measured by a maintained slow resting heart rate.

Louise Hederman, a nursing sister and my future wife, proved a wonderful support while I was in the hospital and gave me devoted care when I returned to Lansdowne Park. She moved into my house then, and remained virtually a permanent resident until we bought a house in Clonskeagh, Dublin, where we both went to live in July 1995, having sold our respective homes. Surgery had one unexpected benefit: it precipitated an early decision by Louise and myself to live together and get married, decisions which have brought us both great joy.

The operation was performed in November 1994. I was restricted during the first three months after surgery by stiffness and limited function, but within six months I had returned to relative normality. I am still conscious of a little discomfort over the hip after vigorous exercise, but I am not restricted by the condition, except slightly in relation to the extension and external rotation of the leg. I could have resumed jogging or light running but I have been reluctant to do so, not because of my new hip but to ensure that my right hip joint remains normal. I would not welcome another hip operation!

I had two further orthopaedic problems. In May 1997, Louise and I spent a holiday in San Diego in California. I had been complaining for the previous year or two of discomfort in the left shoulder joint; this discomfort was episodic and aggravated by such activities as changing gear in the car and certain other movements of the left arm. It was relieved by rest and was not affected by my golf swing. Treatment by rest, injections of cortisone into the joint, and other medication by my physician gave temporary relief but eventually proved ineffective. I was therefore advised by my orthopaedic surgeon to have an operation to remove some osteophytes in the joint. These osteophytes – small, sharp, bony projections found in joints affected by osteoarthritis – were, apparently, impinging on the long head of the biceps tendon, which, according to the ultrasound examination, was being seriously damaged. At the same time, the surgeon could also deal with any other soft-tissue problems which might be identified.

Like any sensible patient, I decided to seek another opinion. I did so first by consulting a second surgeon in Dublin, who was well known for his expertise as an upper-limb surgeon. He confirmed the diagnosis but was less sanguine about the benefits of surgery. My visit to San Diego was partly inspired by my intention to see a surgeon in one of the university hospitals in La Jolla who had been recommended to me as a specialist in shoulder surgery. He confirmed the diagnosis and approved of the proposed surgery; he did so, like the excellent doctor he was, without taking any cognisance of the X-rays or ultrasound results which I had brought with me. The nature of my symptoms, together with a physical examination, was enough to enable him to make the correct diagnosis.

Immediately after my return to Dublin, I entered hospital and had multiple arthroscopies (key-hole surgeries of a joint) to remedy the situation. I was in hospital for two weeks following surgery; during this time, I attended the physiotherapy department each weekday. The surgery appeared to be adequate to deal with the problem, but my symptoms recurred after a few weeks and did not resolve completely for another twelve months. The operation certainly saved my biceps tendon from rupturing. When the symptoms finally resolved, I could not say whether it was the result of the operation, of a three-month period of complete rest of the shoulder undertaken in desperation nine months after surgery, or of some further injections I endured because of my frustration with my poor recovery. In fact, it is likely to have been a combination of all three factors. The symptoms recurred in mild form after the rest period but then resolved completely within a few weeks.

In March 1998, I went on a fortnight's holiday to Orlando, Florida, with Louise, my son Richard and his wife, Caroline. We golfed every day until our fifth day out. On that day, after playing eighteen holes and returning to our villa, I was bending over the boot of our four-wheel-drive when I collapsed with an extremely severe pain in my right knee. I was completely immobilised and had to be helped by my family and a few neighbours into my bed. My kneecap had been displaced downwards and to the right of my leg; the diagnosis was clearly a rupture of part or all of the quadriceps tendon. The quadriceps – the Latin for 'four-headed', referring to the four sites of origin of the muscle in the pelvis, all of which join together to be inserted into the kneecap – is the powerful muscle in front of the thigh which opposes the hamstrings. A partial or complete rupture is rare but, like the much commoner rupture of the Achilles tendon, can occur spontaneously and without any unusual effort or accident. In my case, it was a partial rupture of that component of the quadriceps called the *vastus medialis*. My injury involved the left-sided component of the four muscles.

We phoned a friend of mine who is an orthopaedic surgeon in Dublin. He confirmed the diagnosis and arranged for us to contact an orthopaedic surgeon known to him in Orlando. It was clearly an emergency situation. The following morning I was moved by ambulance to an orthopaedic hospital, where at six in the evening I had an operation which, according to Dr Swartzberg, the young orthopaedic surgeon, resulted in my tendon being 'as good as new'. I spent the rest of the holiday in the villa or in a golf buggy with my leg in a brace sticking out for all to see, and advising my three companions about correcting the many defects in their swings!

My convalescence was slow but satisfactory. I was not greatly disabled, at least in my own home, as the brace with which I was provided was easily detached and only necessary when I was moving around. I wonder how long I would have been hospitalised after such an operation in Ireland. Certainly my discharge from hospital eighteen hours after surgery was not unexpected in the United States and was clearly the right decision. Since 1998, I have felt soreness in my knee, particularly after walking or following a tough round of golf. This soreness is almost certainly caused by a slight anomalous alignment of the kneecap over the lower end of the femur.

I mention these musculoskeletal problems because of the difficulties they pose to many people who wish to maintain a programme of vigorous aerobic exercise. I cannot say whether my hip arthritis and other orthopaedic problems were related to my running or to other activities. Like many other dedicated runners, I ran regularly on tarmacadam and concrete, but I always had good running shoes and dressed appropriately. Despite many years' contact with runners, I was never conscious that hip arthritis or other major orthopaedic injuries were often reported. Pulled muscles, damaged tendons and other soft-tissue injuries are more common among runners, but what aerobic sport worth indulging in is entirely free of drawbacks? Compared to the injuries sustained in modern rugby, and to a lesser extent in soccer, running is the gentlest of sports. With my ectomorphic build, I doubt whether I would survive one game of rugby.

I believe my hip may have been damaged by the rather intense squash I had been accustomed to playing. Squash is a game of twisting motions and sudden acute turns and accelerations; these movements must put a strain on the hips and knees. Whatever the cause, the inconvenience of the operations and their after-effects was a very small price to pay for the benefits I received from playing squash and running. I also have the added compensation that I can still walk briskly, cycle and play to a handicap of sixteen at golf.

The standard of sports-injury diagnosis which prevailed among doctors in the past left much to be desired. This was particularly the case in relation to soft-tissue injuries. In my experience, doctors were inclined to be too restrictive in their advice, despite uncertainty about the underlying problem, and in management of a particular condition they concerned themselves too much with dealing with symptoms rather than seeking causes.

Fortunately, the situation is now changing as more doctors and physiotherapists are specialising in sports injuries, as technological means of identifying changes in soft tissue are emerging, and as further knowledge of the nature of these injuries is being acquired. It is important that you consult a sports-injury specialist when any disability occurs and if your body is not responding to routine medical advice or advice from a physiotherapist. Your doctor, physiotherapist or specialist should be pressed for a definite diagnosis before undertaking a course of treatment.

Rest may be wisely prescribed at times, particularly in the case of pain, but a major change in one's exercise habits should be considered only if the need for such a change is incontrovertible. Physiotherapy in its various forms is clearly valuable in dealing with injuries, but it too should have a rational basis. Too often, physiotherapy is prescribed when the rationale for it may not be clear.

I was always concerned about the negative and nihilistic attitude of some of my colleagues and the media to running and, indeed, to exercise in general. According to one doctor writing in the *Irish Medical News* in the early 1990s, runners are faddist and compulsively push themselves beyond their limits of endurance. He described the expressions of pain and discomfort which he invariably found on the runner's face:

> His face is a deep and dangerous purple. His pot belly hangs down and sways from side to side, evidence of too many good dinners and pints of porter. His thighs are a putty pink and goose-pimpled. The poor fellow probably thinks that he is doing himself some good. He is your quintessential jogger.

Doctors are much less nihilistic about exercise

74

nowadays, almost certainly because of the accumulation of major population studies from many parts of the world which show the lower mortality of people who indulge regularly in aerobic work and leisure exercise. A recent study from heart specialists and epidemiologists in Denmark reflects international findings in this area. The Danish specialists have been studying more than seven thousand adults of both sexes since 1976 and have followed them up to 2000. The men who were active over this period had a mortality of 66 percent compared to those who were deemed to be sedentary, and similar figures were found for the women. Men who were inactive when the study started but who subsequently became active derived the same survival benefit.

The authors showed that exercise had a strong independent effect on health and longevity. Importantly, they confirmed other reports that moderate aerobic exercise – say, walking at a symptom-limited pace for two to four hours per week – was as effective in reducing mortality as more strenuous exercise.

The importance of moderate exercise is mirrored in the Irish Heart Foundation's Slí na Sláinte campaign, which was launched five years ago. The campaign has standardised a system of signage in many of our cities and towns which encourages regular moderate walking exercise in attractive surroundings. It has since been adopted by a number of other national heart foundations worldwide.

Nonetheless, we need more active support from health professionals, particularly doctors, if we are to encourage politicians to recognise that a public policy supporting aerobic exercise and sport in its many forms in the home, in schools and in the community is one of the cheapest and most creative ways of improving public health and reducing binge drinking and crime through the provision of more active and creative opportunities for our young people. We also need a more enlightened policy in our medical schools, where such aspects of public health as exercise, nutrition, smoking and alcohol abuse are neglected and where we still put the emphasis on the treatment of disease rather than its prevention.

In 2003, a faculty of sport and exercise medicine was established in the Royal College of Surgeons in Dublin, headed by Dr Michael Molloy, honorary medical officer to the Irish Rugby Union and a consultant physician in Cork. He will be working closely with the medical profession, providing courses for general practitioners and other doctors in the Royal College and in the medical faculties of the five Irish universities. This augurs well for the future participation of health professionals in encouraging exercise and sport among the population. We doctors need to prescribe more exercise, less abuse of alcohol, avoidance of smoking, cultivation of healthy eating habits and reduced dependence on drugs, both prescribed and illegal. Our new commitment to exercise and sport should help to bring much-needed pressure to bear on our politicians to improve the country's infrastructure of sporting and exercise facilities.

Many doctors, including some orthopaedic surgeons, warn about the adverse effects of running on roads and other hard surfaces. They emphasise the risk of arthritis and other musculoskeletal injuries. While it may seem to be more comfortable to run on softer surfaces, my experience suggests that non-competitive runners are not prone to arthritis unless they have already incurred joint damage, usually as a result of a contact-sports injury during their earlier years, or if they have an abnormal alignment of the legs. Other injuries are also unusual; these are caused by traffic accidents, generally due to the runner's own carelessness, to falls, or to excessively strenuous or inappropriately competitive effort. I saw little evidence of musculoskeletal or cardiovascular ill-effects among the many non-competitive young and middle-aged runners and joggers I encountered during my twenty-four years' running experience. Certainly, the risk of serious injuries among people who play contact sports is much greater than among runners.

This is not to say that runners should not take reasonable precautions to avoid injury and accidents. You should learn to run properly. There are as many running styles as there are golf swings. Do not run on your toes, unless you are a sprinter, and use your arms and body in the most efficient way. If you are a beginner, seek advice about your running style and technique from a sports professional or other seasoned long-distance runner to acquire an optimal method of running. Although you might find you prefer running on tracks or pathways, do not be worried about running on tarmacadam or concrete as long as you have good running shoes. Wear bright clothing at all times and reflective clothing at dusk and at night, and always run facing oncoming traffic. There are many books on jogging and running which the beginner will find useful; details of a few them are given in the bibliography on page 158.

I had this to say about running when I was invited to contribute to the RTÉ programme *Thought for the Day*. My title was 'The Pain of Running':

> Running has become one of the great social activities of our day. Hopefully the sport will endure and remain part of the social scene. It is a non-elitist and inexpensive pastime with many advantages for the participant, not the least being the opportunity to meet and enjoy other people, and to make contact with and develop an awareness of the environment.
>
> The media frequently write rather disparagingly about running and runners – half-seriously, half-jocosely. A familiar comment refers to the look of

pain and discomfort on the runner's face. Only the eccentric or the masochist could voluntarily endure such torture! But here the writer misses the point and the non-running reader may be misled. Running has achieved widespread popularity with normal, sensible people because they gain a sense of fulfilment, a sense of achievement, through the transient discomfort of physical stress.

Longfellow said: 'Know how sublime a thing it is to suffer and be strong.' Perhaps the euphoria some long-distance runners enjoy is a mark of this sublime thing, a sublimation of life's problems and stresses.

We cannot achieve nor can we learn without some sacrifice, and to enjoy we must endure – and perhaps the desire to enjoy without enduring, without suffering, is a root problem in our modern, materialistic society.

Bishop Fulton Sheen, during his famous broadcasts, often spoke about the dangers of self-indulgence. Antichrist would come, talking of peace, prosperity and plenty, and we would seek salvation without the Cross. But there is no joy without suffering. Let the media writers know this when next they look at the runner's face.

*

The better your training and the more you adhere to the 'rules of the road', the less likely you are to suffer from accidents, injuries or other undesirable side effects of jogging or running. Good training is based primarily on adopting a graduated programme which allows for the slow functional adaptation of the body and for the acquisition of an optimum mental approach. To reach full training such a programme may require six months or more, depending on your previous exercise capacity. You may suffer from cramps at the beginning, but these should cause little trouble if you train gradually. They may occur at night, particularly in older trainees, but can be easily prevented by taking a quinine tablet on retiring. (Quinine is better known as a treatment for malaria – formerly called 'Jesuits' bark' after its medicinal value was discovered by the order's missionaries in the cinchona tree bark in Malaysia several centuries ago – but more recently was discovered to affect the nerves controlling muscle.) If you have any doubt about your exercise capacity, you should ask your doctor to arrange an exercise stress test.

I was often asked during my running years about the dangers of running and the possibility of dying during such activity. I wrote several articles on the subject of running- and squash-related deaths in the 1980s; at the time, I had access to a considerable amount of research material on the subject. Running deaths are rare, and most fatalities have been the result of runners being struck by motor vehicles. I have no information about the number of heart attacks and deaths during the popular Dublin and Belfast marathons over the last twenty-five years, but five heart deaths were recorded during the last twenty-three London marathons, in which 550,000 runners participated – an incidence of one death per 110,000 runners. Those with heart disease and heart-disease risk factors are advised not to participate in the marathon without seeking prior medical advice. Nonetheless, in some heart-rehabilitation centres, patients who have recovered from a heart attack are permitted to run in a marathon, as long as they do appropriate training.

From an analysis of figures for many marathons, it was estimated in the early 1980s that roughly one heart attack will be reported for every 100,000 marathon runners and that some of these people recover. It is not surprising that deaths occur among runners when one considers the variety of people of different shapes, ages, motivations and degrees of fitness who enter these events. Extensive research and post-mortem data have shown that it is virtually unknown for a healthy heart to stop during exercise, however vigorous. Victims almost invariably have evidence of heart disease and, except in the very rare case of death in a teenager or of someone in their twenties, they are usually found to have evidence of coronary disease.

In the younger subject, a rare heart-muscle disease called cardiomyopathy or a very rare congenital defect in the conduction system of the heart-controlling mechanism is the likely cause of death. Some of these congenital defects cannot be detected by any known clinical method and would require very sophisticated diagnostic techniques to identify – procedures which would be too complex to apply in routine screening. Even if individuals with rare congenital conditions could be identified, it would not be feasible to examine every person who runs.

You can greatly reduce your risk of a heart attack, however, if you make sure you do not suffer from any of the common risk factors for heart disease: cigarette smoking and uncontrolled high blood cholesterol and high blood pressure. Every adult person, irrespective of their exercise habits – and at least by the age of thirty – should visit their doctor to ensure that they have no obvious heart disease, and that their cholesterol and blood-pressure levels are normal. If these levels are raised, appropriate corrective treatment should be prescribed. The risk of a sudden heart attack in low-risk persons is extremely remote.

In the case of a sudden heart stoppage, the victim could recover with timely and efficient cardio-pulmonary resuscitation (CPR). All ball-game referees and some players should be fully trained in CPR techniques to maintain life while awaiting the arrival of an emergency ambulance equipped with a cardiac defibrillator. A mobile phone should be available to facilitate communication with the emergency services at all competitive sporting events – and the emergency cardiac-ambulance number should be known, at least to the referee and the players.

Other adverse effects and even deaths that occur during running are caused by hypothermia and hyperthermia. I only realised later that I was hypothermic after my first Dublin marathon in 1981, but fortunately, as I mentioned earlier, I was met at the finish by my family, who had been supplied by the organisers of the event with special protective wrapping material, and I responded quickly to re-warming measures. During marathons and half-marathons, in cold weather, you should arrange to be met by a friend or family member with a flask of hot, weak tea at the halfway mark. Long exposure to the cold when running at a slow pace and while wearing little clothing can greatly increase the risk of hypothermia. In these islands, be wary of north and east winds and try to keep to the sheltered side of the road.

In warmer climates, hyperthermia (overheating) is a possible complication of running. The risk is increased by high humidity, direct sunlight and the absence of wind. Unfit and older people who run relatively short distances at a fast pace can be at risk.

My advice about running fatalities conformed to that of all the experts on heart disease and sports injuries. In October 1984, a famous runner in America, Jim Fixx, died while running; his death gave rise to wide international publicity. My interest in exercise and heart disease was well known by then and I was often consulted by the press and radio to explain the need to take sensible precautions before adopting a vigorous aerobic exercise programme. I was aware that Fixx was known to have been a couch potato before he became addicted to running and to have walked no further than to his car. He had been grossly obese and a heavy cigarette smoker before taking up an active lifestyle. He subsequently became one of the great gurus of American running and wrote several best-selling books on the subject, including *The Complete Book of Running* and an annual illustrated diary.

Fixx was reported to have had symptoms of angina for some time before his death, but he had refused to see a doctor. In commenting on his tragic death, I suggested that, if he had not shed his sedentary lifestyle for the running track, he might have died sooner rather later. He lived for twenty-two fulfilling years after he had belatedly taken up running. All major research studies confirm that joggers or runners have a better health record and a lower mortality than sedentary people, even allowing for other risk factors. I avoided all strenuous exercise when I had a cold or flu, or felt unwell for other reasons. I advise others to check with a doctor if they experience symptoms such as chest pain, dizziness or unusual fatigue while running.

Boredom during running, particularly on one's own, is one of the great deterrents for both the novice and the less committed. I too found it a problem initially, but it was one I overcame, as running on my own became a contemplative exercise and a relief from the frenetic activities of my professional life. I also used my brain during running by doing mathematical exercises, such as multiplication or division. I would, say, multiply 356 by 829, and remember the product until I could check the result on my return home. Like the prolonged training required in order to run comfortably, the accuracy of mental computations without pen and paper can be acquired with time and practice. I also used the time to reinforce my memory of poems and other items I had learnt in the past. Thus, I built up a large 'database' of W. B. Yeats's poems, which I started to memorise after my retirement in 1988.

As a result, while I usually ran alone, I was never lonely. We certainly go through life with much unused cerebral capacity: I was astonished at the many empty spaces waiting to be filled in my mind.

There are other answers to boredom. I tried running in different and pleasant places, changing my distance and pace, and challenging my physical fitness and stamina by interval or fartlek running. In this type of running, you cover measured distances at a fast pace, stopping or slowing down during each interval. Such interval running is a valuable addition to training for the competitive runner.

Even now, ten years later, I have not lost my nostalgia for running. When I see a graceful and athletic runner on the streets or the university campus beside my home I have a sudden urge to take off. I also feel a transient moment of sadness – no doubt a subconscious reminder of the passage of time and the inexorable approach of age.

WALKING

Walking is the mainstay of the active elderly person but is beneficial for all age groups. It is an excellent means of maintaining fitness and, like running, is both enjoyable and addictive if we persist with it. As with running, the beginner should adopt a graduated programme of walking. Some stiffness and soreness of the leg muscles is not uncommon in the early stages of such a programme. Many people derive added enjoyment from walking with their spouse, family or friends, by exercising a dog, or by joining a walking or hill-climbing group. You should aim to walk in pleasant surroundings, away from traffic if possible, and safe from predators, human and otherwise. Carry a stick if there are unfriendly dogs around. Keep your eyes on the ground, particularly if the pavement is uneven or broken, and keep your hands out of your pockets in case you have a fall. If you have any tendency to unsteadiness, a stick should be carried.

It is best to rest for a while after meals. I try to do two to four miles on three days of the week, but I would walk more often if I was not already committed to golf and cycling. I walk at a pre-symptomatic pace – that is, at a rate which will make me just conscious of increased breathing, may cause me to perspire a little after a mile or two, and is likely to induce a pleasant feeling of slight muscular fatigue by the time I get home. Walking should not prevent one from maintaining a conversation with a companion. Living as I am in a windy climate, I try to walk in sheltered places on such days. For example, if there is a westerly gale, I tend to walk north or south on the sheltered side of the park or road. Trees, hedges, walls and houses give valuable protection from cold and blustery winds.

It is important to wear proper walking shoes.

They should be comfortable, with suitable non-leather soles and heels. Runners make excellent walking shoes. They have a long life, are not too expensive, and can be worn about the house and garden. New shoes should be broken in gradually. I wear light clothes in the summer, moderately warm clothes in the winter, and a wind-proof jacket when the chill factor is high. Clothing should be loose rather than tight. I never go walking in good or formal clothes; I prefer a tracksuit or an old pair of pants, an old shirt or singlet, and a sweater, particularly if I am inclined to perspire. An old cap or hat is valuable if the day is chilly, as is a comfortable scarf. If you get too warm, the cap and scarf can be carried.

*

We in Dublin are fortunate to have the Dublin and Wicklow Hills so close to us. Indeed, in the whole island of Ireland our mountains and many areas of rugged beauty make a fine backdrop for the hiker and walker. My own house in the Dublin suburb of Clonskeagh is little more than three miles from the nearest hills. I can think of no activity more enjoyable than spending a Saturday or Sunday hill-walking. The wide-open spaces, mountain views, forests, streams and sight of the distant sea bring me close to nature and away from the frenetic urban life of the city. The companionship and sense of fulfilment experienced there – ending with a visit to a local hostelry, happy in front of a fire and with a pint of Guinness in the hand – is as close as one can get in this world to my idea of heaven.

A hill-climb twice a month will lead to a satisfactory degree of fitness but it is an area of recreation which needs to be governed by strict rules. Proper boots and clothing, a compass and a mobile phone, and knowledge of the local topography and weather conditions are minimal requirements. Other essentials are a first-aid kit and a water bottle. Above all, one should never hill-climb alone. For security reasons, there are always at least three of us.

Joining a walking club is a good introduction to hill or country walking. It provides excellent social support, which is particularly important for those of us who are retired and at risk of becoming reclusive. In Ireland you can get full information about walking and walking groups, and about hill and mountain climbing from the Mountaineering Council of Ireland (see page 159). There are also many international rambling and walking organisations that offer organised walks in every corner of the globe. Try Ramblers' Holidays at www.ramblersholidays.co.uk, who offer more than a hundred walking safaris on all six continents.

DANCING AND SWIMMING

Dancing is another form of exercise which is enjoyable and ensures good social integration. Old-style ballroom dancing is particularly appropriate for older people, although the excessively loud amplification which is the rule at public dances is a serious deterrent. This noise pollution is particularly difficult for the elderly because of hearing defects which tend to distort the discordant sounds emanating from the loudspeakers. I was brought up in the tradition of the old-time and slow waltzes, the foxtrot and the more sophisticated rhumba and tango. The cha-cha-cha and the boomps-a-daisy were later and more vigorous variations.

Open-air Irish dancing at the crossroads was popular during my childhood in Dingle in County Kerry in the 1930s. Music was provided by a fiddler and an accordion or melodeon. A dedicated night's dancing at such a function would equal in energy expenditure what would be required to do a fast half-marathon. Set dancing was the rule. 'The Walls of Limerick' and the eight-hand reel were popular and were indulged in with great gusto, in terms of both energy and high-spirited shouting that might raise the roof, if such existed. I can recall no dances in pairs; these were certainly more innocent times. Whether the local curate attended discreetly to ensure good behaviour is not clear, however. More formal dancing by single dancers doing the hornpipe, or groups of trained dancers, was more common at that time in the metropolitan world than it is today, but I cannot recall such formal dancing in Kerry, at least at the crossroads.

The famous film *A Dance Hall of Desire*, which depicted a night in a dance hall in County Mayo, gave little impression of the crossroad dancing in Kerry. While the film provided a good insight into the social mores and

87

the inhibitions of the country people of the west, and the somewhat sordid background of the dance hall, it lacked the exuberance and the spontaneous enthusiasm of the Kerry dances, and the wholesome freshness of the open air. Those nights in the open, often under brilliant starlit skies – no longer seen since darkness left the earth – were hugely enjoyable, despite the fact that little alcohol was part of the scene. At a time when transport was very limited and the houses were widely scattered in the hills and countryside, the dancing, like the Sunday Mass, provided one of the few means of social cohesion.

*

Many people ask about the virtues of swimming as an aerobic exercise. I learned to swim when my children were being taught in their early teens but I draw the line at this activity now, not only because of my sensitivity to cold but also because there is little aerobic benefit from swimming for those who are as incompetent at it as I am. As an aerobic exercise, swimming falls far short of walking, running and ball games in terms of efficiency, except, perhaps for the good or competitive swimmer who covers long distances. It is not a weight-bearing exercise – because of the buoyancy of the water – which reduces its aerobic component. Nonetheless, it is frequently advocated for special purposes, such as the treatment of back and other musculoskeletal problems, or when problems with the feet prevent standing. It does improve flexibility and is of course practised by many as a source of enjoyment.

Swimmers tend to be heavier than most other athletes. I assume that this results from the fact that the swimmer has a greater proportion of fat. Increased subcutaneous fat certainly provides certain advantages for the swimmer. Fat has a lower specific gravity than muscle or bone and is clearly of advantage in providing more buoyancy and perhaps greater speed in competition. It also may act as a form of insulation against the cold.

While swimming is not an ideal aerobic exercise, certainly among simple dippers, there is no reason why it should not be included in an eclectic exercise programme. I suppose that, for the sake of safety, we should all learn to swim or at least to tread water, but this is one of the many counsels of perfection which are easier to propose than to practise. It might be easier to take all sensible precautions to avoid drowning.

CYCLING

I have always been deeply attached to cycling, a mode of transport and a leisure activity which has many advantages and attractions. My impecunious state as a student at University College Dublin from 1939 to 1945 meant that I cycled everywhere on my ancient Raleigh, bought for one pound at a police auction. Almost everybody in college was dependent on the bicycle during and immediately after the war years. I can recall great cohorts of cyclists appearing in the streets of Dublin and at intersections, particularly during rush hour. New bicycle equipment was scarce, but ersatz spare parts and the ingenuity of the repair shops kept things going. Our local repair shop was in a broken-down garage under the Scouts Hall in Richmond Hill close to my home, and many a crisis was averted by Fitzpatrick, proprietor of the shop.

Apart from cycling to and from the boat club during college term, I also had some summer holidays cycling around Ireland. The bicycle was the only feasible way of touring the country. We carried our baggage, camped at night, cooked our own food, and seemed to be unaware of the vagaries of the weather and the rather primitive state of our equipment. Our bikes were decrepit and we had our share of punctures, snapped chain links, and even, on one occasion, a broken crossbar. The machines were heavy, with poor braking and gearing systems. Nevertheless, hardship did not seem to impair our enjoyment, nor did we ever have a serious accident. We did many long and arduous trips at this time, the most strenuous being the 130 miles from Galway to Dublin in eleven and a half hours, with no significant side effects apart from severely excoriated bottoms! What today might seem intolerable hardships were an accepted part of our way of life then. It was a simple, relatively tranquil life, and one where we were almost oblivious of the horrors which were taking place in Germany, Russia and the rest of the world.

In recent years, it was difficult to use my bike regularly and frequently in Dublin because of the hostile environment which existed in the city for the commuting cyclist. The bicycle was an important and ubiquitous form of transport for the community when I was growing up in Dublin in the 1930s and 1940s, and continued to be reasonably popular up to the late 1960s. Before and during World War II, the bicycle and the tram were virtually the only forms of transport, and people appeared on the most primitive and unlikely of machines.

Since 1945, the scene has slowly but dramatically changed. Motor traffic has taken over almost completely. Facilities for the motorist have been extended, at enormous cost in terms of material, spatial and visual resources, while facilities for the cyclist have been at a standstill. One of the most efficient, economical, healthy, sociable and ecologically friendly modes of transport had been ignored and neglected by city authorities and successive governments in favour of the private motor car – the least effective in terms of the economy, the environment and the quality of life of the community.

When I drive or cycle against the heavy traffic in Dublin and see the long lines of slow-moving private cars, occupied in most cases by one person, I have a feeling of despair about the direction the human race is taking. Only the irresponsible can accept the logic of one person commuting in a vehicle which weighs ten times or more his or her weight, and which contributes so much to aerial pollution and to the destruction of the planet's finite resources. It is predicted that the current world count of more than one billion cars will have increased to two billion by 2020. What will posterity, facing the prospect of a serious depletion in world resources and a

91

major loss of diversification in the plant and animal kingdom, think of the arrogance and selfishness of the twentieth-century generations of the Western world? If the conflict between individualism and collectivism continues to be as one-sided as it has been in our time, I have no doubt that future generations will pay dearly for our extravagance and greed.

I have for thirty years or more been sporadically vocal in public about the failure of city and government authorities to include cycling as an integral part of transport policy. In October 1993, I accompanied my brother-in-law and about two hundred other cyclists in a public demonstration through the streets of Dublin, seeking better facilities from Dublin Corporation, as it was then, and the government. Subsequently, in response to an editorial in the *Irish Times*, I wrote the following letter to the editor, which was published:

> Sir, Dublin cyclists will welcome your editorial 'On the Bike' (October 15). However, you say that too often cyclists in Dublin are a careless lot. You suggest that the new Dublin Cycling Campaign Organisation should use its influence to improve the behaviour of cyclists.
>
> While I agree that the behaviour of some cyclists leaves much to be desired, it is unrealistic to think that, under the current unfavourable and under-privileged circumstances which cyclists are exposed to in Dublin, advice from the cycling organisations or any other agency will effect the desired changes in behaviour. Cyclists will conform to the traffic rules and regulations when, and only when, they are treated with the same consideration as motorists and pedestrians. Because of the lack of cycling facilities, there are times when, for personal-safety reasons, the cyclist is obliged to break the law.

The encouragement of cycling as a means of transport and as a leisure activity would have immense economic, social, environmental and health advantages for our city. As such, it would benefit all our citizens, and Dublin would be a more pleasant city to live in. With a fraction of the cost of improving the roads for motor traffic, cycle pathways and bicycle-parking facilities could be provided, and perhaps less ambitious road plans would suffice.

We have wide pathways and, at least in the suburbs, they are often peopled by few pedestrians. At relatively little expense and with a little imagination, we could follow the initiatives of other cities, such as Stockholm and Amsterdam, where footpaths are widely shared by cyclists and pedestrians. And even if economics is the dominant driving force of modern society, I suspect that a viable cycle-pathway system would be at least as effective as an elaborate roadway system designed for motor traffic only.

Cyclists have limited lobbying powers, at least compared to the motor industry. This should not prevent the authorities of this city and country from doing what is best for the whole community.

Happily, the situation in Dublin is changing. I was a member of and medical adviser to the Lord Mayor's Commission on Cycling, established by our 'Green' Lord Mayor and member of the Dáil, Mr John Gormley, in the autumn of 1994. It was a well-chosen group which included representatives of the various organisations and authorities concerned with transportation and social policies in Dublin, as well as cycling interests and a few prominent citizens, including the Church of Ireland Archbishop of Dublin, the Most Reverend Donald Caird, a keen cyclist. The group's report was published in 1995.

Although such reports tend to be quietly shelved, at least in Ireland, considerable progress has since been made in improving facilities for cyclists in Dublin and reducing the dominance of the private motor car. We recommended that cycle pathways be constructed in a radial fashion extending from the city centre to the outer suburbs along all the main thoroughfares. This programme has been partially implemented and, despite the difficulties of imposing such a facility on roads designed for cars and pedestrians only, the cycle lanes have been reasonably successful and appear to have increased the number of cyclists who are commuting. By the end of 2003, 250 kilometres of one-way cycle paths had been completed, costing 20 million, while 57 million has been invested in quality bus corridors which can also accommodate cyclists.

The only adverse comment I have to make about our cycle tracks refers to their occasional poor maintenance by a few of our local authorities. In the course of various public and private works, contractors dig up the tracks and all too often do not return them to their original pristine state. The resultant bumps and depressions make for uncomfortable and possibly dangerous cycling, and the older cyclist, who finds the more solid mountain bike too heavy to use, is particularly disadvantaged. Unless maintenance is properly carried out and roadwork damage to the cycle pathways is immediately and properly repaired, the excellent and innovative programme of cycle paths in Dublin will prove to be a failure.

We also suggested improved facilities for the parking of bikes and for better security. By the end of 2003, 2,500 cycle parking spaces had been provided in the Greater Dublin area by local authorities, and further measures to encourage cycling are being planned by the Dublin Transportation Organisation. A particularly exciting project, the S2S pedestrian and cycling promenade, stretching for 17 kilometres along the Irish Sea coast from Sandycove in the south to Sutton in the north, is now being planned. The project has been approved by the government and local authorities as a new amenity for Dubliners and visitors to the city. Moreover, 2005 will see the transfer of Velo-City, an international cycling conference, from Paris to Dublin, when further plans for traffic integration will be an exciting prospect for all Dublin commuters.

Car-traffic restrictions and new traffic-calming installations are having some influence in reducing the dominance of the motor car and thus making things a little easier for the cyclist and the commuter using public transport. We recommended that new housing estates should be provided with cycle lanes *de novo*, but I believe this recommendation has been largely ignored by the planning authorities. This is particularly unfortunate for our children growing up in these new suburbs. To add to the restrictions on children cycling, the Safety Council of Ireland recently advised parents to discourage their children under twelve years from cycling where there is heavy motor traffic. According to a recent news report, 70 percent of children walked or cycled to school a generation ago, compared with 30 percent today.

Cycling is an ideal aerobic exercise. It enhances cardiovascular fitness and specifically strengthens the leg muscles and particularly the muscles of the quadriceps in the thigh. One has only to see how the muscles in the lower limbs among competitors in the Tour de France are developed. These are the most powerful muscles in the body, and as such they have a vital priming function on the heart, lungs and circulation, contributing to an economy in energy utilisation by the body and to cardio-respiratory fitness. Regular long-distance cycling, particularly of a competitive nature, leads to an increase in mass of the leg muscles in younger people. Even short commuter cycling has been shown to improve muscle power and oxygen consumption. The importance of strong legs becomes apparent as we get older, when many of the premature disabilities associated with ageing are related to weakness and poor coordination of the lower limbs. Despite being in my eighty-first year, I have retained my ability to walk briskly; also, because of the crucial part leg-power plays in golf, I still play to a handicap of sixteen, with little contraction in the length of my tee shots.

Apart from some commuting and leisure cycling around Dublin, I did a number of longer trips around Ireland in the summer in the 1970s and 1980s. These were always with my brother-in-law Thomas Bacon and his rather energetic and athletic daughters. Tommy is a very enthusiastic and fit cyclist and would invariably be ahead of the posse during our long trips. We covered most of the peripheral parts of the country over the years, doing up to sixty miles a day, with each outing extending over four to six days. We would start about nine in the morning, eat a light alfresco lunch, keep up our cycling until five or six in the evening, and then seek a bed-and-breakfast to stay in. We would stop to visit places of interest and we were relatively indifferent to the weather, although I was definitely sensitive to cold; cycling in continuous rain could induce in me an unpleasant degree of hypothermia.

I experienced this unhappy state while cycling on the Dingle peninsula and again while cycling from Waterford to west Cork. Happily I found instant and effective relief in hot whiskey, dispensed in a convenient pub. It was reassuring on these occasions that there is no legislation which would allow the local guards to sustain a charge of drinking an excessive amount of alcohol while being in charge of a bicycle!

Having deposited our panniers in the B&B, and after a bath or shower, we used seek out a local restaurant

96

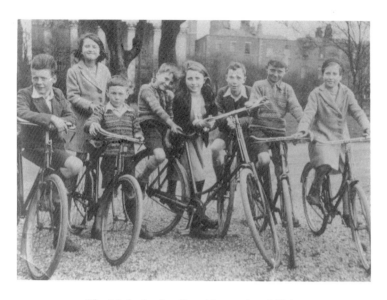

The Mulcahy family with cousins, 1934
The author is second from the right

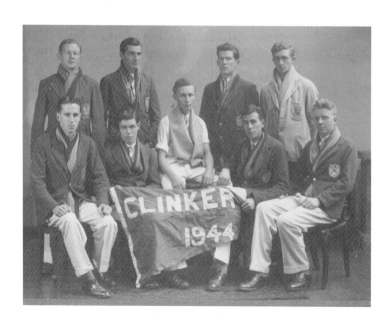

The UCD Junior Eight, 1944
The author (back row, extreme right) rowed No. 2 stroke

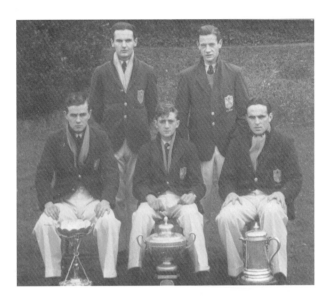

The winning UCD Junior Four, 1941
The author is the cox, centre

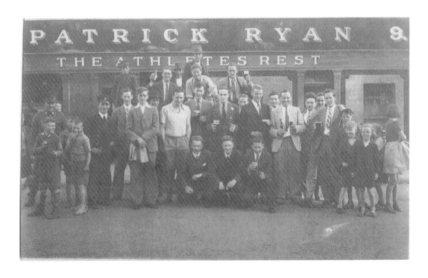

Celebrating after the Metropolitan Regatta, Dublin, 1942
The author is third from left in the main group, holding a scarf

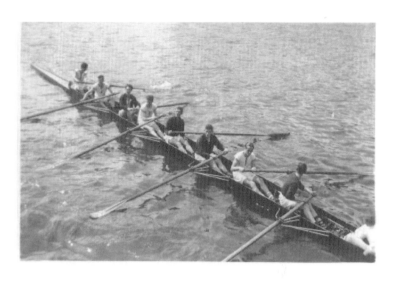

The UCD Senior Eight at the Cork Regatta, 1942
The author is the cox, bottom right corner

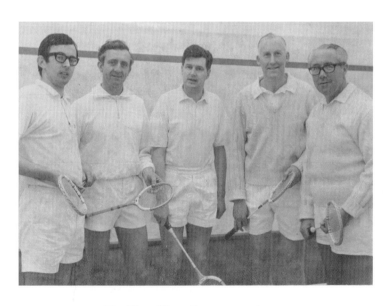

The Fitzwilliam Square squash team,
winners of their section of the league in 1967
Left to right: Peter Piggott, the author, Ken Wall, John Moloney and Con Denver

At the launch of the 'Skipathon' organised by the Irish Heart Foundation, with that year's Rose of Tralee, 1985

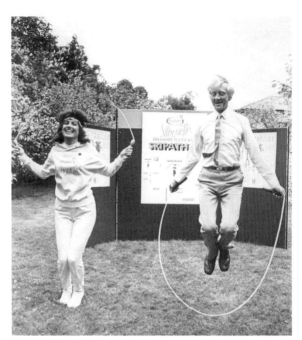

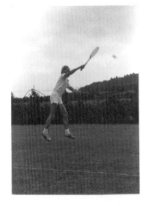

The author playing tennis in the 1970s

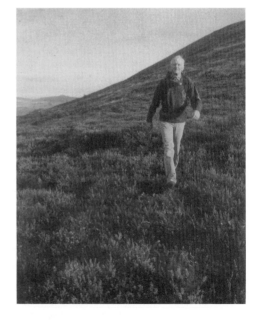

Walking in Glendalough as part of an RTÉ hill-walking programme, 1995

or pub, have a well-deserved pint of Guinness and a meal, and be in bed before midnight. Despite having had several such outings, we failed to find a B&B on only one occasion, in Castletownberehaven in west Cork. Without exception, the B&Bs were excellent: clean, inexpensive and with a high degree of Irish hospitality. The breakfasts were invariably copious and excellent, and in many cases second helpings of sausages, bacon, and eggs were pressed on us by the woman of the house, who was anxious to see that we were well fortified for the next leg of our journey.

One of the pleasures of these cycle trips was meeting the families, and particularly the mother, the *bean an tí*, who presided over the establishment, and whose friendship and hospitality were a constant reminder that much of the old tradition of hospitality and generosity which was an integral part of the Irish native culture could still be found in every part of the country. I include here the North of Ireland, where we did a memorable trip in the summer of 1986 after we had completed the one-day hundred-and-three-mile Dublin-to-Belfast leg of the maracycle.

There was an element of hardship in some of our cycling outings that was reminiscent of my marathons and earlier rowing days. I recall the extreme fatigue and discomfort in my legs while cycling the last twenty-five to thirty miles of our Dublin-to-Belfast maracycle, with a cold and persistent north-east headwind, and with little protection from its baleful influence on the wide main road we were travelling. But I also recall the wonderful relief and the euphoria I felt on arrival in Belfast as I stretched out on the grass in the warm sunshine outside City Hall, as I felt the pleasant fatigue of my stretched leg muscles as they relaxed in recovery, as the sweat died slowly on my warming body, and as I gratefully consumed the sandwiches and champagne which Michael

Scott, our northern host, had prepared for us.

I experienced the same fatigue and discomfort during the prolonged climb of the Vee in the Knockmealdowns in 1990. After travelling through parts of south Tipperary, including a climb from Tipperary town into the Glen of Aherlow, we were pressing into an unpleasant south-easterly as we climbed the interminable Vee on our way to the other side of the Knockmealdowns. On this occasion, severe cramps obliged me to stop at Lismore. By the time I got to the top of the Vee, the cramps were persistent and severe, and involved both my thighs and calf muscles. I was unable to do any further cycling, but fortunately the long descent into Lismore was continuous and I was able to freewheel the entire way. Here I was glad to get into my sister Neilli's four-wheel-drive with my bicycle to finish the journey.

Cycling through the countryside is a most enjoyable pastime, and was a feature of visits my wife, Louise, and I paid to the west of Ireland in later years. We carried our bikes on a specially designed carrier which is attached to the tow bar of the car. We greatly enjoy the fresh air, the easy view of the countryside and the scenery, and the satisfaction to be derived from physical exercise. The only two deterrents are a strong headwind and heavy motor traffic, the first because it is difficult to enjoy the sense of physical freedom and the appreciation of one's surroundings if one has to push hard and keep the head down, and the second because of the feeling of insecurity created by the proximity of heavy traffic, and the unpleasant grinding noise and pollution produced by passing trucks and cars.

We are fortunate that we can benefit from the great advances made since World War II in bicycle technology and equipment, and in the clothing and other personal items designed for the cyclist. My mountain bike, with its twenty-one gears (surely a *richesse*!) and efficient gear-changing system, excellent braking, built-in lock and carrier system, computer, wide tyres and light but sturdy frame, was a joy to ride around the city and for short country runs, but it is now too heavy for my ageing limbs. My thirty-year-old Raleigh racer still seems as light as a feather. It has twelve gears and is ideal for long country runs as well as city commuting. With occasional full servicing by my local bike shop, it should survive to be treasured by a new owner. The problems, so evident during my younger days, of punctures and broken chains and poor or absent gearing, of inadequate braking systems and of heavy and cumbersome frames, are things of the past.

The equipment available now, the excellent carrying systems, the more efficient lighting and braking, the built-in reflectors, the automatic pedal grips, the built-in locks, the tiny computers and various other gadgets, as well as the constantly improving designs, add to the efficiency, safety and enjoyment of cycling. I would urge the would-be cyclist to invest in a good bicycle suitable for his or her age, physical capacity, aspirations and circumstances. I would also advise full investment in suitable equipment and clothing for all types of weather and to maintain visibility at night as well as during the day.. You need a good-quality and secure lock and must always leave the bike in a secure place. Above all, you must adhere strictly to the rules of the road.

I have a greater interest and pride in my bikes than in my car. If I ever had the misfortune to suffer a theft, I would prefer to lose my car than my bike. I would opt for cycling rather than motoring if I had to forego one or other form of transport, and I would depend on taxis or on family or friends to provide motor transport when necessary.

Cycling is undoubtedly the most efficient form of urban transport in economic and ecological terms. It is also more efficient in terms of speed, at least for city commuting. When cycling is encouraged, everyone benefits – even including motorists, as a result of the fact that there is less four-wheeled traffic on our roads. Cycling is also more desirable socially, in that it encourages communication with other people, while the car tends to isolate us, even from our next-door neighbours. Cycling is healthy – and safe, if proper facilities and training are provided by the city authorities, and cyclists obey the rules of the road. As well as offering physical benefits – physical fitness and the prevention of diseases associated with lack of exercise – cycling also has psychological benefits, all of which contribute to a better quality of life.

The failure of city and government authorities, at least up to recently, to encourage cycling as a means of commuting has been unacceptable; the situation is still far from satisfactory. Correspondence in the newspapers, where cyclists, motorists and pedestrians indulge in blame and recriminations, looks set to continue until the cyclist is given equal rights to others. Only then will cyclists adhere fully to the rule of the road. As well as the urban hazards facing cyclists, the narrow country roads are almost bereft of cycling facilities and subject to an ever-increasing volume of motor traffic. Sadly, cycling in the countryside is now dangerous because of the narrow roads and the heavy motor and truck traffic.

Accidents to cyclists are frequent; we have had a few fatalities in Dublin in recent years. Research in the United States has confirmed that 80 percent of cycling accidents are the fault of the cyclist who does not observe the rule of the road. The same certainly pertains in Ireland. Ignoring traffic lights, travelling without lights and proper reflective clothing, not using clear signals when changing course, weaving in traffic and not dismounting when a significant obstruction is reached, are all too frequent here and are obvious causes of accidents.

Helmets are rarely worn and, while there is still some controversy about their value, I know of two serious accidents, one fatal, which almost certainly would not have occurred if helmets had been worn. Toe clips are valuable for long-distance and competitive cycling but are probably best avoided in the urban setting because they may impede prompt dismounting in an emergency situation.

We need a public-education campaign to improve cycling behaviour. That, as well as more consideration by the authorities for the cycling fraternity, would add to the popularity of cycling as a means of commuting and leisure enjoyment.

INDOOR EXERCISE

Indoor exercise in a gym or health centre has become a widely practised form of exercise in recent years. The Greater Dublin area, with a population of close to one and a half million, has at least fifty health centres with professionally trained staff and a wide variety of training equipment and swimming facilities. These facilities are also available, often in equal degree, countrywide and in many of our leading tourist and commercial hotels. Health centres are mostly utilised by the better-educated, probably because of their greater interest in health promotion and because of the fairly substantial costs involved.

Some equipment in the health centres is designed to encourage isometric exercise aimed at enhancing muscle mass and strength. While a modicum of this form of exercise is suitable for the middle-aged and older person, heavy and sustained isometric work should be reserved for younger people who want to increase muscle mass and strength.

Equipment designed for isotonic or aerobic exercise and training is aimed at cardio-respiratory fitness and improved musculoskeletal function and flexibility. This equipment, which includes treadmills, bicycle ergometers and rowing machines, can be used by all age groups, but the same rules about the need for graduated training must be observed.

To achieve a satisfactory degree of fitness, I usually recommend that this form of exercise should be practised three times a week, and, with short breaks, for an hour each session at 75 to 80 percent of maximum heart rate during peak exercise. Fast walking would be equivalent to 70 to 75 percent of maximum heart rate. You should seek the advice of the professional staff at such

centres if you need more guidance about your programme.

The benefits of health-centre training, in terms of
fitness, flexibility and function, can be equally achieved
with home exercises, and at a much reduced cost, however. I have been doing simple calisthenic exercises on
and off at home for many years to maintain flexibility,
and I have a good-quality bicycle ergometer which I use
when I have neglected my cycling. The ergometer helps
to maintain the strength and suppleness of the leg muscles and to retain my cardio-respiratory fitness. The dis-
advantage of home exercises is that motivation is perhaps
more difficult to maintain over the long term than when
under the supervision – and availing of the advice – of
health-centre staff.

Twenty minutes on a bicycle ergometer three or
four times weekly should be sufficient to ensure optimum
leg function and a modicum of cardio-respiratory fitness.
You should start each session at a relatively low resistance
and gradually increase this to the point where you will
find yourself perspiring at the end of the session. A treadmill can also be used. I have had no experience of a rowing machine but this offers the added advantage of providing benefit to the arm, shoulder and back muscles.

There are a number of books available about
home-flexibility programmes. My programme is a simple
one: it lasts not more than ten to twelve minutes per session and is often performed with music in the background. While standing, I can carry out various movements of the arms and shoulders: rotation at the shoulder
joints, and extension of the arms to the front, back and
outwards. I can do similar movements of the neck and
back – extension in all directions, and rotation – but am
careful to avoid excessive movements which might damage ligaments and the discs between the vertebrae.
Movement should never be forced, should always be

within the limits of comfort and normal function, and should be pain-free.

Lying prone or supine on a towel on the floor, you can exercise the abdominal and leg muscles. Again, this should be done within the limits of comfort. In the supine position, raising the head and shoulders to the vertical position will strengthen the abdominal muscles. Lifting and holding the leg for about five seconds, knee flexion and extension, and ankle rotation will benefit the leg muscles and joints. Again, all these activities should be graduated at the early stages and should never be a cause of pain or discomfort.

Stretching exercises are popular today, particularly among runners and football players. There are various simple ways of stretching the thigh and leg muscles, although I have found it difficult to maintain these exercises regularly during my running career. I believe that it requires a special commitment to continue doing them, I suppose because of boredom and being uncertain about their value. As stretching exercises are believed to reduce the risk of pulled or torn muscle, many sports professionals recommend them before running or competitive ball games and during the recovery period. I think I would have adhered more to their practice if I was convinced of this.

Any of the following exercise programmes should provide an excellent degreee of fitness: one hour three or four times a week in an indoor gym or at home, with an emphasis on aerobic exercise for the older person; jogging for forty to fifty minutes four times weekly; walking for fifty to sixty minutes four times weekly; or cycling about fifty miles a week. The inclusion of a variety of other exercises aimed at enjoyment, relaxation, social cohesion and long-term involvement, such as football, golf, tennis and squash, will help to provide the spice of variety and may be of aerobic value.

GOLF

My exercise history would be incomplete without a reference to golf. My parents lived near the inner-city golf club, Milltown, and were associated with it from 1927. They were late starters and played the game purely for pleasure. It provided gentle exercise and recreation during their later years. It also gave my father an opportunity to meet and talk to some of his old political friends, many of whom were also members of the club.

I joined Milltown Golf Club in 1939 as a university member, shortly after my brother Padraig and sister Elisabet had joined as junior and university members, respectively. We were more competitive than our parents and the three of us have been closely connected with the club ever since. Padraig was captain in 1964 and later president and a trustee of the club. Elisabet was the lady captain in 1974, while I was captain in 1954, at the early age of thirty-one. I am also a member of Portmarnock, where I play my winter golf.

I have never thought of golf as a recreation aimed at achieving fitness. It is too leisurely and interrupted an activity to be of any great aerobic value unless one moves quickly, as can be done if playing with one other person and with a clear course. Golf does, however, contribute to flexibility and to slowing the attrition of the musculoskeletal system. It is an immensely enjoyable pastime in social terms, and is particularly important for myself and my many colleagues who have reached retirement age and who might otherwise yield to the reclusive temptations of our age group. The contacts one makes at the golf club lead to social activities outside as well as within the club, and permit one to maintain friendships which might otherwise atrophy.

Another advantage of golf is the mental challenge

which is inherent in the game. Like all ball games, your attitude and motivation largely determine how well you play and how you succeed in competitions and in match-play. I started playing when I was seventeen years and achieved a handicap of seven about fifty years ago, although I was never particularly competitive at that time. By 1968, when I stopped playing for a spell of twenty years, I could play reasonably well. Yet, like all amateurs, I was inconsistent, sometimes playing within my handicap, at other times – and more often than not – having an untidy, erratic round with too few pars over the eighteen holes.

Golf poses a major personal challenge because I know that I will play well if I adopt a positive, aggressive attitude to the game. I will play badly if I am negative, defeatist and think only of what can go wrong with my shots. It is a maxim of the game that, if you think you are going to win and your approach is positive and confident, you will play well and be far more likely to win. If you have doubts about yourself, if you are negative and pay too much attention to your opponent's game and too little to your own, you are lost. No matter how badly your opponent plays, you will often play that much worse!

Golf is such a personal challenge that it will cause men of confirmed maturity and professional standing to behave like bad-tempered children. If they fail to overcome the challenge of the game, it upsets their ego and shatters their self-esteem. If they have a particularly successful round, on the other hand, they will preen like peacocks, full of good humour and confidence, happy that they have reached the ranks of the professionals in terms of future performance, and only reluctantly – and then patronisingly – aware of their opponents. No business, professional or other success compares in importance to that rare event, the immaculate round of golf, the occasion when one plays one's 'usual game'. I know because

I am one of them! One of the problems we amateurs face is that we do not respond to the challenge that performance is based more on our attitude than on our physical prowess.

I pride myself on having a good insight into the golfer's dilemma. I know that I must adopt a positive, aggressive approach to the game. I also know that I must practise regularly, not to improve my swing or my technique, but to inspire confidence in myself through greater familiarity with the game. I might have an occasional lesson from a professional to iron out any faults which may insidiously affect my swing. But fundamentally, a lesson from a professional for a long-standing player like myself is, like practising, mainly beneficial because it enhances confidence.

I do not follow my own precepts, however. I do none of the right things. As I know that putting is the vital factor in good scoring – you drive for show and putt for dough, as they say – I bring my putter home to practise on the hall carpet but seldom follow through with the intention. More often than not, I forget to bring the putter when I next go out to play!

An accurate short game around the green is the next most important factor after putting. I am full of good intentions to practise this short game but I seldom do so, despite having access to excellent facilities. No doubt I shall continue as I am doing, fantasising about the day when I will play like a professional.

After twenty years' spent running, playing squash and having a busy professional life, I returned to active golf in 1989, after I had retired. I was surprised to find little deterioration in my game in terms of accuracy and length. I also found a degree of confidence and a positive psychological approach to the game which I had largely lacked in earlier years. I tried hard to be more positive and aggressive, and to think always in terms of winning.

I would try to visualise Pete Sampras, Andre Agassi and Martina Hingis and how their tennis seemed to be inspired by pressure – and how they had the courage to respond in such a positive way. Why could I not do the same? After all, I assume that I have the same cognitive faculties as they.

I was greatly helped by doing more practice when I resumed in 1989. Ten days of intensive practice at the Club Méditerranée in the Algarve in 1991, where there are excellent golfing facilities, was a great fillip, and resulted in my winning several competitions during the following year. My confidence was undoubtedly helped by my physical fitness, an advantage I did not enjoy during my previous golfing career. It was also helped by reading *Golf Is Not a Game of Perfect* by Dr Bob Rotella, a well-known sports psychologist and adviser to many leading golf professionals. Unless you are a person of extraordinary self-confidence, I would recommend that you read it.

I have won more golf competitions and matches during the last twelve years than I won during my first thirty years, when I was younger but also less fit and less aware of the need to adopt a positive approach to the game. When I am under pressure now, I grit my teeth and try to force myself into positive thinking. Driving myself relentlessly might have the same effect, but I have no doubt that my physical fitness makes a major contribution to the physical and psychological aspects of these successes.

PART III

ADVICE ON EXERCISE

EXERCISE AND AGEING

Ageing is inevitably associated in our minds with the approach of death. In the last ten years or so, because I am now in my eighty-second year, I think more of my forthcoming demise, but I have accepted the prospect philosophically and as a natural part of life. The fact that I do not believe in a world hereafter does not influence my attitude, nor does it make me less spiritual. Natural death after a long and healthy life should be a cause for celebration. 'In balance with this life, this death', in the words of Yeats. Perhaps the oldest person to die in Ireland in recent years was Brigid Dirreen, whose age was 109 years. I had visited her two years before in Galway, where she was pleased to meet me again, having been my nanny during my first year in Dublin at the time of the Civil War.

One of my main concerns now is the quality of my final years. The biological lifespan of *Homo sapiens* is fixed and has been unchanged since the beginning of recorded time. Living in a perfect environment and avoiding all harmful lifestyle habits, it is likely that a person's normal lifespan is around ninety years, with some scatter from eighty to a hundred, with a few people over a hundred. We are all familiar with the Methusalah story of nine hundred years in the Bible and the more recent claims made of people living to a hundred and fifty years or more, but all such claims have been made in primitive societies where no birth or mortality statistics are available. It is also well known that very old people tend to exaggerate their ages. Despite extensive research by demographers and anthropologists in these remote areas where such old people are reputed to live, none of these claims have been confirmed.

In Western countries such as Ireland, how far away are we from achieving a normal lifespan? This gap can be estimated by our life expectancy, a term which is used to define the average length of life at various ages from birth upwards. Life expectancy is based on the census preceding its measurement; it establishes the length of time in years and months when half of each age group will have died. It can be measured for the entire population, for men and women separately, and for different social and occupational groups, depending on the information provided by the latest census.

In Ireland the last census was in 2002 but the life tables are not yet available. Based on the life tables derived from the previous census in 1996, life expectancy from birth was seventy-three years for men and seventy-eight years for women – a far cry from our normal lifespan – but, in view of the continued fall in heart and stroke mortality since 1996, I expect an improvement when the latest figures, based on the 2002 census, are available. The raw data derived from the 2002 census show a 16 percent increase in the number of people in the country who are eighty-five years and over, a finding which is consistent with the anticipated improvement in life expectancy.

As in most other countries, Irish women have a better life expectancy, not because of an inherently longer lifespan but because of their healthier lifestyles. This situation may change, however, as women adopt more 'male' habits in contemporary society. A measure of this trend is the rising incidence of lung cancer, due to smoking, in women in Ireland at a time when the male incidence of the disease is falling.

Life expectancy at birth has been increasing gradually since the census commenced in Ireland (then part of the United Kingdom) in the mid-nineteenth century. It was as low as forty years at that time. The increase has accelerated in the last fifty or sixty years, mainly because of the huge fall in infant mortality. If life expectancy is measured at fifty years or more, however, the improvement is much less dramatic because so many preventable deaths still occur in the middle-aged. The attached illustration shows in graphic form the life-expectancy situation in the United States during the last 150 years.

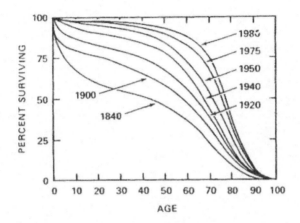

US sequential survival curves,1840 to 1980. Note the change in
the shape of the curve as infant mortality declines
(US Bureau of Health Statistics)

The American experience closely reflects that of Ireland and Britain. In the early years, many infants died at birth and many others died young from the effects of epidemic diseases such as tuberculosis, diphtheria, pneumonia and poliomyelitis. Such deaths are now rare, so that the graph shows a tendency to squaring over the years. Most deaths in those under thirty years are caused by accidents, violence or suicide.

113

In an ideal society, with the total elimination of disease, this graph should show a squaring, with a relatively straight line to the late seventies or early eighties and then a precipitate drop at ninety to a hundred years.

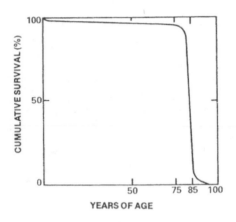

The rectangular survival curve

The squaring of the life pattern is unlikely to be achieved in its entirety, because of the vagaries of human behaviour and the inevitability of major disasters, but it should be the target of a rational society.

We can measure ageing in chronological terms but we also need to measure the various physical and cognitive manifestations of ageing. Some of these cannot be altered or influenced, but others can be modified by our habits and lifetime behaviour. The table on the following page gives details of these.

CONDITION	LIFESTYLE CHANGES
Cardiac reserve	Exercise, not smoking
Dental decay	Dental care, diet
Metabolism of glucose	Weight control, exercise, diet
Hearing	Noise avoidance
Intelligence	Training, practice
Memory	Training, practice
Osteoporosis	Weight-bearing exercise, diet
Physical endurance	Exercise
Lung function	Exercise, not smoking
Reaction time	Training, practice
Blood cholesterol	Diet, exercise, weight control
Social cohesion	Behaviour, practice
Skin health	Sun avoidance
Blood pressure	Salt limitation, weight control, exercise

Due to the great improvement in our health, particularly during the last fifty years, we are faced with an increasing proportion of retired and elderly people. It is estimated that by 2020 the number of people over seventy years will have doubled in Ireland. The proportion of retired people to working people will change from one in five to two in five; we know that the number of people over eighty-five years increased by 16 percent between 1996 and 2002. Hence the worry about pension funds and the prospect of fewer people having to support an increasing population of retired and disabled people.

The widely prevalent diseases and disabilities of the middle-aged and the elderly are the result of the lifestyle adopted by a prosperous and self-indulgent society where raising the standard of living in terms of acquisitions is the chief objective of the government and those who elect it. Unhealthy eating, lack of exercise, smoking, excessive intake of alcohol, violence and risk-taking now largely account for the gap between lifespan and life expectancy. These habits in middle life result in many premature deaths and leave many old people with long-standing and chronic disabilities which condemn them to dependence on society and the overburdened health service. Unless increased longevity is accompanied by good health, the demands on health services will continue to grow beyond our resources. For instance, in recent years, the cost of the health service in Ireland has been increasing at four times the increase in inflation, from 2 billion in 1994 to an estimated 10 billion in 2004, and it is unlikely to stop there.

The health services in this and all other Western countries are in a state of chronic crisis because of funding shortages; I see little likelihood of this situation being remedied in the near future. Unlimited funds would be needed to satisfy an increasingly demanding and litigious public and an ever more expensive health service. There are several reasons for this situation. These include the rapid expansion in high technology in diagnosis and treatment, and the decreasing cost-effectiveness of high-tech medicine, where too much emphasis is put on tests and too little on the clinical approach, which includes history-taking and patient examination. Other reasons are the increase in the use and cost of drugs, pressures from the medical industries, the failure of the medical profession to keep abreast of drug technology and take cost efficiencies into account in their practice, and the professional and administrative costs resulting from litigation. Above all, there is the exponential cost of treating older people.

Fifty or more years ago, most people with a terminal illness died within a few days, and not infrequently without medical intervention. Nowadays, thanks to

116

developments in medical and surgical care, prolonged illness and disability are the rule, and are becoming more common because of our ageing population. Chronic illness in the elderly is rarely subject to cure, and many such patients are liable to frequent readmission to expensive hospitals, and to hospitalisation for prolonged periods.

The dilemma for our health services is created by the conjunction of the recent expansion in high-tech medicine and an increasing and ageing population. Many older people are the victims of chronic disease caused by earlier unhealthy lifestyles. But the onset of disease in the elderly is not inevitable. With optimum health during life, death may come as a natural end because of gradual cellular failure, a gradual loss of function which is part of growing old. When we are old, our health and independence are largely determined by our earlier habits and motivations. The worsening crisis in the health service will not be solved until two fundamental cultural changes take place in our society.

Firstly, we must individually and collectively take more responsibility for our own health. The medical professions and the government must give a higher priority to public-health education and to an environment which is conducive to healthy living.

Secondly, because health-care resources exist within certain boundaries which at the same time have to be consistent with efficiency, we must accept limits on the treatment of the chronic, intractable, incurable and progressive illnesses experienced by the old. Should old and terminally ill patients occupy many of the beds in our acute health care and expensive hospitals? How can we best deal with this very difficult ethical problem? Should we continue antibiotics and chemotherapy in patients with progressive and terminal disease, and with a poor quality of life? Should we resuscitate patients with terminal disease if they suffer a sudden heart stoppage?

Unfortunately, medical professionals hold widely different views on these matters and I can see little prospect of establishing an agreed policy, at least among doctors. There should be a clear public-health policy on this issue. In the context of today's more compassionate society, we can hardly give higher priority to those who have adopted healthier lifestyles.

There is little we can do to counteract ageing and the final dissolution of the body, nor can we hope to cure the chronic diseases and diminishing functions which precede dissolution. Although old people are increasingly exposed to advances in diagnostic techniques and therapeutic interventions which may confer some benefit, too often inappropriate treatment may prolong life without adding to the person's quality of life. Indeed, the individual's quality of life may be adversely affected because of prolonged and repeated medical or surgical treatment, hospitalisation, and alienation from family, friends and familiar surroundings. Too often we see old people – who should enjoy the support of family and friends in a domestic or appropriate institutional background and should face a dignified and natural end – subjected to multiple medications, to uncomfortable and not infrequently useless interventions, and to the loneliness and humiliation of being away from family and in the presence of strangers. This is what that great social philosopher and controversialist Ivan Illich called 'the intensive care of the dying'. When the end is at last reached, it comes as a relief for the patient's family and friends, who have witnessed the prolonged suffering of their loved one, as well as for the patient.

With the anticipated increase in the proportion of older people in this country, it is imperative for reasons of humanity as well as the funding of our health services that stricter control of medications for the old and a more balanced and compassionate approach to medical interventions should be observed by the medical profession and by other health professionals. As our organs deteriorate with age, our tolerance of drugs is reduced. This is not always appreciated by those dealing with the elderly and is a further reason to adopt a conservative approach to using medication. Polypharmacy, where patients are on multiple drugs, is a circumstance which can be found too often in the elderly. It not infrequently leads to apathy, depression, confusion and proneness to accidents.

There is currently much research taking place to identify an ageing gene or genes in an attempt to extend the human lifespan through genetic engineering, but it is not certain that such a gene exists. It is likely that ageing and a limited lifespan is a result of failure of the human cell (except cancer cells) to survive beyond a certain fixed limit. To extend the human lifespan to a hundred and fifty years or more would create a nightmare when added to the current population explosion, which is contributing so much to poverty, refugee movements and a deteriorating environment.

Ageing, leading to death, varies in its progress from one person to another. There may be a genetic factor which accounts for such variability but the freedom from harmful lifestyles and environmental factors, and the consequent freedom from disease, ensures that the attrition of ageing is reduced to a natural or physiological level, with a deterioration in function of about 1 percent every year, starting in the mid or late twenties. A lifestyle which extends survival also ensures a life of health and independence during old age and a shortened period of disability and dependency before the end. Those who are younger should remember that our earlier habits and motivations are the bedrock of an active old age.

My own concern is to live an independent, physically and mentally active, and enjoyable life as long as I can, and to avoid a prolonged period of dependency, despair and depression at the end of my days. This can be done by remaining physically and mentally active, by continuing to take a creative interest in affairs, and by maintaining social contacts. It is natural to lose influence and even the attention of others as one retires from the corridors of power and as one's friends and contemporaries pass gradually from the scene, but it is unnatural to resent such changes after an active and productive life.

There is substantial evidence that those people who are most adapted to the ups and downs of life, who accept adversity with a certain equanimity and success with a measure of humility, and who possess a sense of humour and a feeling of collegiality and community, have better physical and psychological health. Marcus Aurelius, the Roman emperor of the first century, was perhaps the most famous of the Stoics. His *Meditations* provided much of the high-minded morality of the Victorian era and have been a great inspiration for me during my lifetime. He did not speak of God but believed in the godliness of virtue; included in the concept of virtue was love and the acceptance of adversity with resignation. Aurelius wrote that we should always love our brethren, even our enemies, and should accept pain and pleasure with the same detachment. Although these injunctions are both tall orders, the Stoics, who predated Christianity, and their philosophy of virtue, provided the basis of Christian morality. I have no doubt that an understanding of human nature and a tolerance of the failings of others, combined with a philosophical outlook on life and death, contribute to an equable state of mind, which adds to a healthier life in physical and mental terms. Successful ageing is based on spiritual, as well as physical and mental, attributes.

In Western society, ageing is associated too often with a negative stereotype. Other more traditional societies have a different view of the aged, attributing to them wisdom and a link with tradition and the past. In such societies, the old continue as part of the extended family. Until they become totally dependent on others for their needs, they continue to play an active role, with certain defined responsibilities. Recent research has shown that old people, even those confined to an institution, if they are given certain duties and responsibilities consistent with their ability, and particularly if they are given some part in decision-making, remain healthier, both physically and mentally, and need not conform to the stereotype which prevails in Western society. Nor do old people necessarily welcome the co-dependency provided by our voluntary and social services. Many will prefer to remain independent of others as long as they are capable of looking after themselves.

Ageing and retirement are closely related events in one's life. I am often asked about the desirability of a medical check-up by imminent retirees, particularly if they wish to adopt a more active exercise programme. It is, of course, important that such a person should be aware of any potential health problem or disability, but it is equally important that older people should not become victims of over-medicalisation, as can happen if the significance of some clinical finding, such as marginally raised blood pressure, recurring colds, or a trivial symptom is exaggerated. It is an unfortunate fact that the elderly in Western countries are too often subjected to excessive medicalisation, particularly in the use of drugs, and that the treatment may prove to be the primary factor in perpetuating their symptoms and leading to chronic dependency on the doctor. We should question the necessity of medications, particularly in the elderly, and in people who are prescribed multiple drugs and where normal health appears to be restored.

There are many symptoms that are common among older people and that, as part of the natural process of ageing, are not related to disease, nor do they require complex or prolonged medical intervention. An older person may complain of various aches, joint pains and stiffness, particularly in the morning. These symptoms may be wrongly attributed to significant arthritis. They are best treated by a proper balance of exercise and rest, however, and by very simple pain-reducing remedies when necessary.

In my experience it is not unusual for those in the eighties or more to complain of minor bouts of angina or of neurological symptoms which we call transient ischaemic attacks and which sometimes presage a stroke. These symptoms may lead to more significant complications but this is by no means always the case. Even if we contemplate the worse scenario, however, it is highly unlikely that we can bring about a 'cure' in the very old. Conservative treatment and tender loving care may prove to be the most humane and effective approach. Admission to hospital, with its consequences of intensive investigation and treatment, and of separation from family and friends, is too often counter-productive in terms of the subject's physical and emotional wellbeing.

Diminished production of enzymes and other secretions may lead to dry mouth, dry eyes and increasing flatulence. Eye drops are effective in relieving dry eyes. Sucking a boiled sweet or taking a little lemon or orange juice will relieve a dry mouth, which commonly occurs at night in bed. Excessive flatulence can be managed by avoiding too much high-fibre food and red meat. Other foods which are poorly tolerated can be identified by exclusion trials. The exclusion of these foods may improve digestion.

Older people tend to spend more time in bed but to sleep less. Sleep patterns are often disturbed, with frequent waking and dreaming. Poor sleep can be associated with daytime napping and fatigue. It may be aggravated by a sleeping partner, by unsuitable bedding, lighting or noise, by bad eating and drinking habits, and by irregular hours being kept. Mood changes, including depression, may also be a factor. Adopting regular sleeping habits, avoiding fluid intake for a few hours before retiring, and avoiding late stimulants, such as alcohol and the caffeine contained in tea and coffee, should help. A quiet house, subdued lighting and spending a few tranquil hours before retiring will also help improve sleeping patterns.

We do not require as much sleep as we get older. For those in their seventies and beyond, five or six hours of continuous or interrupted sleep should be compatible with normal health. The principal problem doctors encounter is the anxiety of those who believe that lack of sleep is harmful to health. Sensible explanation and reassurance will assuage anxiety and may improve the length and quality of sleep. An occasional or regular mild sleeping tablet may be required, particularly to assist falling asleep, and a mild pain-relieving tablet, such as paracetamol or aspirin, taken once or twice a day, will help the scattered aches and pains experienced by the elderly.

We tend to become a little more anxious with age, and we may lose some confidence in situations which previously caused us no bother. Going into town to the cinema or to a concert can be undertaken without any difficulty by the young or middle-aged, but the elderly may be a little apprehensive about the prospect of such simple tasks as parking and arriving in time. It is important to plan our activities carefully by allowing enough time for them and by foreseeing possible difficulties. The frequency of mislaying items such as keys, glasses and handbags is more often caused by inattention while laying them down rather than to a defective memory. Neither are young people immune from this problem. In dealing with such minor frustrations, the trouble can be avoided by adopting a regular drill when leaving things down in the house.

During my many years spent counselling patients who had recovered from a heart attack, I always raised the question among male patients of their future sexual activity. It was very unusual for a patient to touch on the subject, because of the traditional modesty of the average Irish male and his reluctance to discuss such a personal matter, even with a doctor. Once the issue had been raised by me, some people expressed no interest in sex or said they had no opportunity for sexual activity, but others, even the more elderly, were grateful for the opportunity to explore this important aspect of rehabilitation after illness.

Poor erectile function has been the main obstacle to a successful sex life in elderly males, but the introduction of sildenafil (Viagra) about five years ago has made an important difference to the late-middle-aged or elderly men who frequently suffer from this complaint. Viagra has also been effective in younger men who have suffered from organic or anxiety problems which affect erectile function. Other drugs with the same or similar actions are now available or are being developed; these may contribute further to this important improvement in the lives of older people. Affected people should contact their doctor for advice on erectile function or can call a confidential medical information service at 1800 633 363 (provided courtesy of Pfizer, who manufacture Viagra).

Sexual problems among women are mainly caused by dyspareunia (discomfort during sexual intercourse), lack of arousal – because of poor understanding on the part of one or both partners – or simply aversion to sex. Doctors have little experience of managing such complaints, which are best dealt with by trained sex counsellors.

It was traditional to discourage patients with

heart disease from taking part in sexual activity, but during my many years of counselling such patients I found no reason to believe that such activity is likely to have any adverse effects. Indeed, bearing in mind the importance of sex in the lives of some elderly people, doctors need to be more proactive in broaching the subject when the opportunity arises.

It is generally believed that memory deteriorates with age. While there is undoubtedly some attrition in cognitive skills, in line with reduction in physical functions, it is clear that most people as they age do not use their cognitive functions to the full. Tests of memory, intelligence and IQ show that, with appropriate training progammes, considerable improvement in these functions can be achieved in people in their eighth decade and later. Such improvement is enhanced among the elderly who retain a sense of independence, responsibility and social cohesion.

A good means of training and testing your memory is to do a crossword regularly. In recent years I have been doing this. I find my mind is not quite as flexible as it used to be, but the deterioration is relatively marginal and does not prevent me from helping – and being helped by – other crossword aficionados.

A check-up is desirable at retirement. This should consist of a simple clinical examination by your doctor, with a carefully taken previous medical history. Blood pressure and weight should also be measured. Routine tests are not required, apart from a cholesterol profile or any test which may elucidate a clinical problem which might arise. Even the cholesterol test can be ignored if you follow a healthy diet and do not have a strong family history of heart disease. Apart from the cholesterol test, the necessity for other screening tests, such as breast and prostate screening, is controversial and should be left to the discretion of the examining doctor. If your doctor suggests further tests or referral to a colleague for further examination, you should ensure that you understand the reasons for such action.

Whatever health check is provided, in the final analysis adherence to a healthy lifestyle, combined with a sensible approach to exercise and continued participation in hobbies, interests and social affairs, must be the bedrock of our approach to successful retirement and to the enjoyment of our later years.

The elderly have most to gain from regular aerobic exercise: mobility, independence, vitality and confidence, better coordination, muscle and bone strength, social integration and a reduced risk of the mood changes often seen in old people. We should remain as active as possible both physically and mentally, into old age, but this ideal can only be achieved by adapting oneself to the inevitable restrictions of the ageing process. As far as walking and jogging are concerned, it is necessary to start slowly as we grow older if we are to achieve a comfortable second or third wind, and to get into a comfortable rhythm of movement. As we approach the critical threshold of three score years and ten, coordination begins to deteriorate and reflexes become less efficient. It is therefore important to avoid injury and to keep your wits about you when close to motor and cycle traffic.

When I reached my mid-seventies, I began to feel minor musculoskeletal symptoms, such as muscle soreness and stiffness, particularly in the early morning. These generally resolve as soon as I am up and about, and have completed a few simple calisthenic exercises. I am sometimes asked if I feel my age. I think I have become more conscious of my age in latter years, not only because of these early-morning aches but also because of my clearly lessening exercise capacity and flexibility.

Up to my early or mid-seventies, when asked if I felt my age, I would respond that I felt no different than I had when in my twenties. My recent experience conforms to the well-documented evidence that physical prowess, flexibility and stamina begin to deteriorate along a semi-exponential curve at some stage in the seventies. This is well illustrated by the graph of times of marathon record holders for the different age groups: the age of seventy marks a cut-off point between the slow attrition of performance associated with healthy ageing before this date and the quickening deterioration which follows.

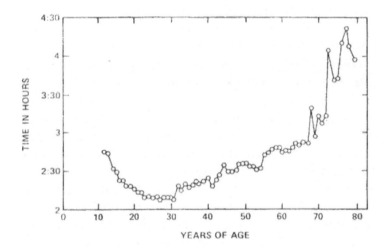

World record marathon times for males aged 10 to 79
(Based on data from *Runner's World* magazine)

Perhaps the biblical three score years and ten refers to this change in our physical prowess and not necessarily to our demise! This natural change in exercise capacity need cause no concern, however, as long as we adapt sensibly to such limitations.

Despite the increased attrition which we can

expect in our seventies and later, I find that regular and sensible exercise is even more important to me now than in the past. It has protected me from the social isolation which is not uncommon when one is retired, and which can be associated with such mood changes as depression and feelings of loneliness and isolation. For instance, the Tuesday four-ball in Portmarnock with my regular friends – including the traditional visit to the nineteenth hole – is something I always look forward to. A good walk or cycle is followed by a welcome sense of relaxation and even mild euphoria, counteracting the ennui one feels if confined indoors for too long.

I still maintain an eclectic approach to exercise. This includes walking three to four miles three times weekly, cycling, playing golf and doing simple home calisthenics. Since I stopped running, my resting heart rate had risen from about forty-five per minute to about fifty-six, suggesting a slight diminution in my state of fitness. The resting pulse rate is the simplest and one of the most reliable indices of cardiovascular fitness. You can check it by feeling the radial or femoral pulse about ten or fifteen minutes after retiring to bed, and without the recent consumption of stimulants or any other cause of sympathetic stimulation. This pulse is easily found by gentle pressure of the index and middle finger close to the wrist or in the groin when lying down. The maximum heart rate I can reach with full exertion during a stress test is now substantially less than formerly, but this is a normal consequence of age and does not impair my ability – or need – to continue being aerobically active.

I had neglected calisthenic exercises in the latter days of my running but I resumed them recently. These exercises are simple aerobic movements which, to relieve boredom, can be done to music. They are mainly designed to exercise the abdominal, leg and shoulder muscles. The exercises, if performed regularly and systematically, are valuable in slowing the deterioration of the body's flexibility and strength. Care must be taken, however, to avoid increasing joint mobility beyond physiological limits. Otherwise, injuries can result. I am particularly careful to avoid excessive spinal movements, as these may damage the apophyseal joints, which connect contiguous vertebral bones, or damage the discs between the vertebrae.

You will find books on calisthenics and aerobics in the health and sports sections of your local bookshop. Work out a programme which will suit you and which is aimed at maintaining flexibility and rhythm. You can get advice about these exercises from a gym instructor or a physiotherapist.

I ask myself if we are designed by nature or God to continue in good health right up to final dissolution from old age. I believe most of us are, if we lead a healthy lifestyle free from the ravages of cigarette smoking, excessive alcohol intake, unhealthy eating habits and a sedentary life. Such a healthy life is often equated with a hairshirt existence, but the opposite is in fact the case. Using your body and mind, adopting a modern, healthy and varied cuisine, and drinking in moderation (or not at all) will add to your quality of life, not take from it. With such a lifestyle, the great majority of people should enjoy active and creative lives up to or close to the biological lifespan of ninety years, and more than a few may pass this limit.

This advice about smoking, alcohol and healthy eating aims to allow you to reach a normal lifespan, as well as improving your quality of life. Much is written about healthy eating but it requires no detailed advice to achieve such an objective. Simply follow certain principles: no food is bad but the red meats and high-fat dairy foods should be eaten in moderation. Adding salt freely to food and eating very salty foods are best avoided because excess salt can raise blood pressure in some people and is related to stomach cancer. Vegetables, fruit and salads are the basis of healthy eating, and the more the better. While high-fibre foods are healthy and often recommended by nutritionists, the older person should be aware of the side effects of eating too much fibre. We become less tolerant of fibre as we age and we may suffer from abdominal discomfort and excessive flatulence if we indulge too much in these foods.

Fish and other foods low in saturated fat are freely available, and pastas, potatoes and other starchy foods are permitted unless you have a weight problem. We should eat less when we get older and it is wise to eat the main meal of the day at lunchtime or early in the evening. Sleep tends to be easier and more settled after the digestive functions have finished. Fluid intake should not be excessive for a few hours before retiring.

Can we overdo exercise? The answer is yes, at least for the elderly; overdoing it is a possible cause of injury in the older person. In a recent report about the active elderly, it was shown that 70 percent of injuries could be attributed to excessive enthusiasm when adopting an exercise programme. The commonest types of accidents involve the knees, calf muscles, Achilles tendons and shoulder joints. It is important therefore not to take too obsessional an approach to exercise and not to proceed too quickly. Also, we should keep our wits about us when out of doors, just as we should be careful to avoid accidents in the home. Keep an eye out for uneven footpaths and for steps and other obstacles, and keep your hands free and not in your pockets when walking. Tripping over carpets, falling down stairs and other common mishaps in the home are preventable with a little care and attention.

Seventy people, mostly the elderly, died in the Republic in 2001 as a result of falls down stairs. Some were inebriated but others were not. The elderly should be careful to watch their step, and to hold on to the banisters or to have it close to hand. Glasses for reading or bifocals should not be worn on the stairs, nor should awkward objects be carried.

How do we know if we are taking too much exercise? The answer is that we cannot do too much if we listen to our bodies. Clearly any stressful symptom, such as pain, undue fatigue or breathlessness, dizziness and feeling faint cannot be ignored. But it is wise to exercise regularly and to remain in a constant state of training. Just as in younger people, if we have been sedentary and start doing things too quickly or too vigorously, we may become discouraged or suffer injury. It will take longer for the older person to acquire a training effect. We must therefore be patient in the early stages; given such patience, it is never too late to start. Long-term compliance with a training regime will be assured if we adopt the type of exercise which we enjoy and if we walk in safe and pleasant surroundings.

Dizziness is frequently caused in the elderly when they stand up suddenly. The arteries become a little more rigid and less flexible as we get older, and blood-pressure control becomes more sluggish. The dizziness is caused by a transient drop in blood pressure. The elderly are advised not to stand up suddenly from a sitting or lying position, particularly if they have been resting for a long period. Such dizziness does not indicate a propensity to stroke or heart attack. If dizziness is frequent or severe, however, and not simply caused by postural change, it should be investigated by a doctor.

What type of exercise should be advocated for the late-middle-aged and the elderly? My answer would be any form of exercise which you enjoy and which suits your inclinations and circumstances. An eclectic programme of exercise is ideal. While I would give walking

131

pride of place for outdoors and dancing for indoors as suitable forms of exercise for the elderly, I would also encourage other forms of activity. This is important if, for example, circumstances are such that you cannot go walking because of bad weather, a cold or an injury. It is here that indoor exercises can be useful and enjoyable to maintain all-round flexibility. Simple calisthenic exercises will maintain flexibility, while fifteen minutes on a bicycle ergometer or walking machine is good for heart and lung function and maintains leg-muscle strength and coordination. As we survive into the seventies and eighties, impairment of leg strength and coordination may first cause a significant disability and lead to accidents. Swimming, cycling (in safe places and obeying the traffic laws!), golf and other non-strenuous ball games are other alternatives.

At least I am trying to practise what I preach to others: that regular active exercise is a major contributory factor to growing old gracefully. It prolongs our independence, preserves our physical attributes and postpones the disabilities associated with ageing. Regular exercise enhances a good quality of life, and has useful psychological effects which counteract depression, anxiety and mood problems, which are all too common in older people. Exercise should, however, be combined with regular rest periods. One to two hours' rest in the afternoon is hugely beneficial in order to strike a balance between all our physiological functions.

Nowadays, 99 percent of children are born healthy in Ireland and Britain; with few exceptions, they remain healthy into adult life. The principal causes of disability and death in children and young adults are accidents, violence and suicide. As we approach middle life, however, serious illnesses appear and their prevalence increases. These illnesses include heart disease, stroke, cancer, bronchitis, emphysema, diabetes, arthritis and many other less common conditions. The sedentary are afflicted by the prevalence of premature ageing in their sixties and seventies, brought on by these conditions, many of which are irreversible and disabling.

Is the prevalence of these chronic diseases in the middle-aged and the elderly the norm, or are we designed by nature to continue in good health right up to final dissolution from old age? This is a fundamental question which we must answer if we are to give proper guidance to people about healthy living and about achieving a normal lifespan.

It seems to me that we were intended to live healthy lives up to old age but that a number of factors in our environment, and particularly in our personal behaviour and diet, contribute to the high prevalence of chronic disease in the middle-aged, and thus to the major disabilities we find in older people. With increasing knowledge derived from worldwide medical research, we are well on our way to identifying the causes of these chronic diseases.

Already, we know that coronary heart disease, the greatest scourge among adult people in the Western world today, has its basis in unhealthy eating habits, cigarette smoking and high blood pressure. We know some of the lifestyle factors which predispose to high blood pressure. We are aware of the causes of bronchitis and emphysema, and of several forms of cancers, and particularly lung cancer, and we know what predisposes to diabetes. We also know that physical deterioration occurs more quickly in those of us who are sedentary compared to those who are physically more active. The adage 'if you don't use it, you'll lose it' applies to all the organs of the body, including the mind, and applies to the elderly as well as to the young.

The bony vertebral column in the dry skeleton seen in the anatomy museum is strikingly different in its configuration from the vertebral column of a healthy middle-aged adult. Its pronounced curvature in the upper chest region and its shortening is the result of the absence of the rubber-like collagenous discs between the vertebrae. The pliable intervertebral discs allow the easy mobility of the living vertebral column, and account for our greater height when we are young. The ageing or elderly person tends to show a configuration which simulates the configuration of the bony skeleton, but this tendency is considerably influenced by the subject's exercise habits. Atrophy and thinning of the discs proceeds more quickly in the sedentary ageing person.

In my own case, although I have shortened by about four centimetres since I was fully grown at twenty, my posture has hardly changed despite my eighty-one years, a feature which I attribute to the regular and eclectic exercise programme which I have followed for the past forty years. It is also likely that the apophyseal joints, which permit spinal mobility but at the same time act as stabilising agents between contiguous vertebrae, maintain a greater flexibility in the active person. The natural loss of the spinal-muscle fibres which is part of ageing will be slowed by remaining physically active.

The physically active and physically fit person of seventy years will have the same heart, lung and musculoskeletal function as the person of fifty who is sedentary. The former retains optimum muscle strength, bone density, joint mobility and flexibility.

What should be the ultimate objective of a rational society? Firstly, it should be to live in harmony with nature. The great Russian physiologist Ivan P. Pavlov defined health as a state of being in equilibrium with nature. Certainly, the health of future generations is dependent on harmony with nature, a fact which should compel current generations to avoid nemesis by ensuring that we care for nature as assiduously as we care for ourselves. Unfortunately, the world is in denial about our abuse of nature and the environment, and the effects of the population explosion.

Secondly, we should strive to live lives of high quality, good health and longevity with, at most, only a short period of disability and loss of independence before the end. Exercise plays a vital part in achieving these aspirations. Combined with good nutrition, freedom from tobacco and excess alcohol, accident prevention, and education, we could surely square the survival curve of the human population (see graph on page 114).

In the past we had high infant mortality combined with endemic contagious infections and, not infrequently, epidemics ravaging whole populations. There was widespread poverty and destitution, with accompanying adverse effects on health and longevity. We had little personal control of ill-health in these earlier years. By the second half of the twentieth century, the contagious infections had been largely brought under control and, at least in the Western world, the influence of poverty and destitution was lessening in relation to ill-health.

We now have an epidemic of chronic diseases such as coronary disease, stroke, cancer, diabetes and obesity. These are diseases of affluence and disuse, and are largely self-inflicted. Nearly all aspects of personal and family health, quality of life and longevity are under our own control. It is clear therefore that, in an ideal world, most of us could live high-quality lives up to or close to the end of our biological lifespan.

It is true that health education in recent years has had considerable success in reducing the incidence of stroke, heart attack and other chronic conditions. These benefits have not reached all parts of Irish society to the same degree, however. In both Ireland and Britain, where demographic findings are similar, professional and better-educated people have a substantially better health record and life expectancy than the unskilled and the disadvantaged. In Britain, the mortality of the unskilled is three times greater at sixty-five years than that of professional people, and we probably have the same experience in Ireland. This disparity has nothing to do with genes: it is at least partly due to the failure of the less-educated to respond to health advice about smoking, alcohol, nutrition and accident-avoidance, as has been noted in many population surveys, although there may be other occupational factors to account for the disparity.

Our recent Celtic Tiger period of prosperity was celebrated by reduced taxation and a burgeoning increase in cars, holidays and second homes while relatively little was done to provide the institutions and social services required to care for the disadvantaged and the elderly which should be a moral imperative in any prosperous Christian society. I am inclined to believe the adage that the poor will always be with us, but in any modern, prosperous country, poverty, whether or not self-induced, should be alleviated by society where possible.

HEART HEALTH

The epidemic of coronary heart disease reached its peak in the late 1950s and early 1960s in Ireland and the Western world. The epidemic has been slowly waning in Ireland and all other Western countries since about 1970 but coronary disease is still one of the greatest – if not the greatest – cause of premature mortality in most of these countries. As the figures show, Ireland is lagging behind the other eleven original partners in the European Union, although our figures are gradually converging towards those of other countries.

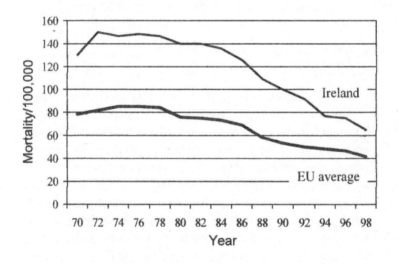

Mortality from coronary disease in Ireland and the EU among men aged 0 to 64 years, 1970-98
(*Ireland's Changing Heart*, 2003)

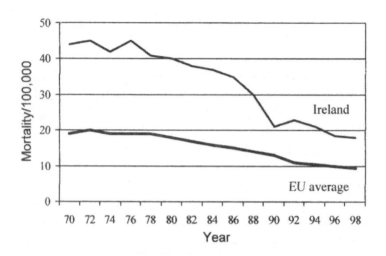

Mortality from coronary disease in Ireland and the EU
among women aged 0 to 64 years, 1970-98
(*Ireland's Changing Heart*, 2003)

During the six years following 1996 there was a
further fall in coronary mortality of 19 percent in men and
15 percent in women in Ireland and a continued conver-
gence towards the rates among our partners in Europe.
This is a significant drop in mortality from one of the
great killers in modern Western society, and we can now
anticipate with greater optimism that current measures to
control the disease will be effective. These include not
only the medical and surgical treatments available in
many sophisticated centres in our hospitals but also the
effects of prevention by changing the lifestyle of the population, including those already afflicted by heart disease.

In 1961, a special heart unit was established by
myself and some of my colleagues at St Vincent's
Hospital in Dublin to deal with the problem of heart disease in Ireland. We had no reliable information at the time

about the cause or causes of the epidemic, nor had we any effective way of treating those who were afflicted by the disease. As we had no means of controlling the epidemic, we were initially helpless in preventing the many sudden deaths which occurred daily both inside the hospital and in the wider community.

We therefore made a virtue of necessity and began to study the background of our patients in an effort to determine the cause or causes of the disease. Within three years, we could reliably report that there was a high prevalence of cigarette smoking among our patients. We identified a similar prevalance of high blood pressure and high blood cholesterol, findings which were being reported at the same time from research in the United States.

So began my lifetime interest in the treatment and prevention of coronary heart disease, not only in patients but also among the public at large. My interest in this area was expressed through the Irish Heart Foundation, which was established in 1966 and of which I was the first president. It was at this time that I became actively involved in a public-health campaign on smoking, healthy eating and exercise. In 1965, we set up a rehabilitation programme for our hospital patients who had recovered from a heart attack. It had been the rule in the past to advise patients after recovery to cease all exercise – in the unsubstantiated belief that such a policy would avoid further attacks – and it was commonplace to stop patients from returning to work, particularly work of a physical nature. Fortunately, not all patients followed this advice.

We started gingerly to turn this conservative approach on its head by encouraging patients to get out of bed when their symptoms had resolved. Instead of the traditional approach of keeping patients in bed for weeks and of discouraging all movement, we encouraged earlier movement, ward activity and earlier discharge from hospital.

Within a year or two, we could confidently advise patients to leave hospital within a week, unless there were complications, and on discharge to adopt a graduated exercise programme that led, within a few months, to them walking up to twenty-one miles a week. Many of these patients were followed by us annually and some were still reporting to us as recently as 2003. Many became addicted to their walking programme and enjoyed better health and a greater sense of confidence in themselves as a consequence. With few exceptions, they were encouraged to return early rather than late to their former employment.

We first reported these results at the World Congress of Cardiology in London in 1970 and later that year in the *Scandinavian Journal of Rehabilitation Medicine*. We noted that 90 percent of our patients under sixty years had returned to work, compared with only 40 percent reported by other doctors – as confirmed by the statistics published at the time by the Irish Department of Social Welfare. In 1970, even among the relatively few cardiologists attending the Congress who were concerned with the rehabilitation of heart patients, the approach in terms of exercise and work was still very conservative. Inevitably our results were received with incredulity and, no doubt covertly, with scepticism. Much of our work in this area is reported in my books *The Long-term Care of the Coronary Patient* and *Beat Heart Disease*.

Patients were also advised about the control of other risk factors. This included advice about healthy eating and strict admonitions to stop smoking. Subsequently, our research was to show that stopping smoking proved to be the single most effective way of reducing the risk of further heart attacks.

Our interest in heart-disease prevention led to the setting up of a department of preventive medicine and health promotion at St Vincent's Hospital in 1970.

Professor Noel Hickey, of St Vincent's, and Professor Geoffrey Bourke of University College Dublin joined me in this initiative. It was the first such department in any hospital in these islands.

We have had departments of preventive medicine in the universities for many years but these have traditionally been staffed by non-clinical doctors and professors – academics who have no direct contact with patients. Such departments have had little influence over the years with practising doctors, although they have played an important role in researching and encouraging various public-health measures and in expanding the social services. Unfortunately, few hospitals still have such departments because of the profession's almost total commitment to diagnosis and treatment, although there has been an encouraging advance in the Health Promoting Hospitals movement in this country and in Europe. Another encouraging feature of hospital practice is the expansion of the cardiac rehabilitation services in all our larger hospitals. These services are largely staffed by nurse specialists and other medical personnel, including nutritionists, physiotherapists and social workers.

In general, the medical profession has had a negative attitude to health promotion and disease prevention. This has been evident throughout the history of medicine. With few exceptions, doctors have concerned themselves solely with the diagnosis and treatment of disease and injuries. More than once in our history, we have demonstrated opposition to important public health measures because they were perceived to be interfering with our professional hegemony. This indifference to health promotion was reflected until very recently in our undergraduate and post-graduate education programmes. As an adverse lifestyle plays a dominant part in causing common preventable diseases, prevention holds far greater promise for the development of a healthy society

141

than even the most advanced medical or surgical treatment. Nonetheless, prevention is still a neglected area. An American population study showed that 75 percent of premature deaths were related to lifestyle or environmental factors. This is surely a challenge to the government and the medical profession. On the other hand, there is now greater evidence of a commitment to health promotion from doctors, the government and voluntary agencies.

Hippocrates, the father of medicine, included healthy living habits in his recommendations. Despite our commitment as doctors to the Hippocratic tradition, the profession is only now grasping the importance of seeking causes for diseases and proffering appropriate lifestyle advice.

It was becoming clear as a result of research both in Ireland and at an international level that sedentary people were more prone to heart disease and that there was no basis for the highly conservative traditional prohibition on exercise. Since then, incontrovertible evidence has accrued that exercise is beneficial for heart patients in terms of health and longevity, if such exercise is properly prescribed. It is clear that active people are less prone to coronary disease. Many recent trials have also shown that regular aerobic exercise improves the outlook for those who have already suffered from the disease. This benefit is independent of other interventions, and the intensity of exercise need not be more than that provided by moderate regular walking. Our prescription of walking twenty-one miles a week or three miles a day is ideal, provided it can be done without distress from breathlessness or pain. This type of programme is now widely prescribed in cardiac-rehabilitation programmes in this country and elsewhere, although a less time-consuming ten to twelve miles a week would be more practical for some and would be highly effective in heart patients as well as in those who are healthy.

A regular exercise programme leading to cardio-vascular and respiratory fitness has the same effect in reducing or getting rid of the pain on walking which occurs in patients suffering from angina as beta blockers, which are acknowledged to be the best drugs for treating such patients. Regular exercise is at least as effective in improving heart function. Combined with appropriate advice about such risk factors as smoking, high blood pressure, obesity and high cholesterol levels, most patients will respond by losing their symptoms, by avoid-ing heart surgery and by reducing their risk of further coronary trouble. Many doctors do not appreciate the importance of offering such a regime to their patients before proceeding to surgery and other more inconven-ient, more expensive and more invasive interventions. The same need to exercise and to control risk factors exists even after surgery or balloon angioplasty (a proce-dure involving the insertion of a tube with an inflatable balloon which can open a blockage in a coronary artery or stretch a partial blockage).

Coronary artery surgery and balloon angioplasty are helpful in selected cases but are only palliative proce-dures. They treat symptoms rather than the underlying cause of the patient's problem, the disease affecting the coronary arteries. Without tackling the risk factors, the patient will still be prone to recurrence of angina or fur-ther heart attack, even after surgery. The best medical practice must seek and eliminate causes, an approach which is not always followed by patients – nor indeed is its importance always underlined by doctors.

The same may be said about patients who suffer from disease of the leg arteries. This common condition is called peripheral vascular disease and is commonly relat-ed to cigarette smoking. It may lead to serious disability and eventually, if neglected, to partial or complete amputation because of loss of blood supply to the limb. The condition will respond to graduated exercise if the patient also stops smoking; in such cases the symptoms will improve and not infrequently resolve completely. Only the exceptional case should require surgery. It is a disease which will rarely be encountered when the habit of smoking cigarettes is confined to our cultural history.

In the late 1960s, I published a leaflet, entitled *Walking to Health,* which gave detailed advice to patients about the virtues of walking and how to follow a safe and enjoyable programme. As a source of information, it was a useful adjunct to the advice given to patients by our rehabilitation team. By the early 1970s, the Irish Heart Foundation had launched a public-health programme advocating more exercise in the pursuit of health and greater political involvement in providing adequate exercise facilities in the country. I and my colleague Professor Noel Hickey represented Ireland at various international conferences dealing with exercise and public policies organised by WHO and the European Community, as well as the European and International Societies of Cardiology. Despite the fact that such activity has been pursued at an international level for thirty years or more, Western society has been slow to take action to reduce the increasing prevalence of obesity, diabetes, heart disease and the other hypokinetic diseases where the benefits of aerobic exercise are largely known.

While it is true that, until recent years, the medical profession was slow to encourage exercise for patients with coronary disease, there were some notable exceptions. One such was William Stokes, the Irish physician who attended the Meath Hospital in the mid-nineteenth century and who was renowned for his teaching and his textbook *Diseases of the Heart and Aorta,* published in 1852.

When writing about fatty disease of the heart, his term for coronary disease, he states:

> We must train the patient gradually but steadily to the giving up of all luxurious habits. He must adopt early hours, and pursue a system of graduated muscular exercises; and it will often happen that, after perseverance in this system, the patient will be enabled to take an amount of exercise with pleasure and advantage . . . The symptoms of debility of the heart are often removable by a regulated course of gymnastics or by pedestrian exercise, often in mountainous countries, such as Switzerland, or the Highlands of Scotland or of Ireland.

Unfortunately, Dr Stokes's advice fell on deaf ears during the ensuing century. Samuel Johnson, in his biography of Jonathan Swift, refers to Swift's belief that his 'grievous malady' failed to respond to his native air in Ireland but 'he thought exercise of great necessity, and used to run half a mile up and down hill every two hours.' Ulick O'Connor spoke to me of Swift's habit of running up and down the stairs in the Deanery, with a servant at the bottom to record the number of times he did so.

EXERCISE TESTING

I supervise an exercise stress-testing laboratory at the Charlemont Clinic in Dublin. Most hospitals and medical clinics provide exercise-testing facilities; this is an essential service in all institutions that deal with heart patients. The testing is performed on a treadmill or bicycle ergometer. We always follow a standard protocol which provides us with valuable information about the subject's fitness and about changes in the coronary circulation, heart-muscle function and heart rhythm which may not be apparent in the electrocardiogram performed at rest. The stress procedure is an essential test in diagnosing angina and related changes in the heart muscle in patients who are suspected of having coronary heart disease. It may also help in deciding whether other tests are required before arranging the most appropriate treatment for these patients.

Exercise testing will provide valuable information not only about diagnosis and treatment but also about long-term prognosis. Certain refinements are provided in the more sophisticated medical centres to improve precision in diagnosis, while sports physiologists in the more sophisticated sports institutions may use other refinements to test the fitness of – and the progress achieved by – more serious athletes. If you wish to commence an exercise programme, a maximum exercise test will give baseline information about your exercise capacity and fitness. Repeat testing can be a good measure of progress, although it is hardly necessary except to please the more introspective or inquisitive. Indeed, your resting pulse will give basic information about fitness as long as you are not on special medication which affects the heart rate.

If you intend to start an exercise programme or to increase your current activities, it is advisable to have an exercise test if you are over forty years of age, in order to ensure that you do not suffer from early heart disease. It is, however, fundamental to health and safety that you are free from the well-known risk factors for coronary disease: cigarette smoking, high cholesterol and blood pressure, and poorly controlled diabetes. It is vital that you have a check-up to exclude these conditions before starting training. Nowadays, diabetes and abnormalities in blood pressure and cholesterol can be easily controlled, so that you can undertake any reasonable exercise and training.

It should be emphasised that you ought to start an exercise programme gradually, whether it is walking, jogging or running, particularly if you are making other changes in your lifestyle, such as stopping smoking or changing your eating habits. A gradual approach will also reduce your risk of injury. It will take a few months of patient, graduated work before you find yourself in a comfortable rhythm and with the confidence to know that you are exercising at an enjoyable level, conscious perhaps of your breathing and of the tension in your muscles, but feeling comfortable and free from any distress. By then you may reach a point where it will be easy for you to keep up your exercise as a lifetime pursuit. You may find yourself addicted to exercise so that you feel deprived if you miss your outings for more than a day or two. Following a long-term exercise regime is not easy but, with proper initial training, many people reach the point where it becomes a key part of their daily lives.

Unfortunately, over the long term, exercise poses major problems for sports and physical-exercise instructors. An intervening illness, an injury, a holiday, a family crisis or simply bad weather may lead to the need to suspend activity and to a loss of motivation. Boredom during walking or running, unsuitable surroundings, unsuitable equipment, an absence of suitable companions, and fam-

Practical Suggestions

The major causes of serious and recurring illness and mortality in our society are cigarette smoking, alcohol and drug abuse, high blood pressure, lack of exercise, unhealthy eating leading to obesity and serious metabolic problems such as abnormal blood cholesterol. In the young, accidents, violence and suicide are the most frequent causes of mortality. We should, as individuals, parents, teachers and health professionals, focus as much on health promotion and prevention as we do on the active treatment of chronic and intractable disease.

The following principles need to be adopted if we are to achieve a life of good quality, health and longevity:

Regular Exercise

1   Remember that aerobic exercise forms the basis of good physical and psychological health, and is as important for an eighty-year-old person as for an eighteen-year-old

2   Check with your GP before beginning any new exercise programme if you are a middle-aged or older person. This is particularly important for older people

3   Take moderate exercise for half an hour each day if you can

4   Do something you enjoy, as you are then more likely to engage in this activity regularly

5   Build an exercise programme into your daily routine

6   Remember that even simple activities such as walking up and down stairs or walking to the shops rather than taking the bus are useful additions to an exercise programme

7   Take comfort from the fact that exercise, in the long term, becomes increasingly enjoyable and addictive

DIET

1   A healthy diet is a well-balanced diet. With the variety of ethnic dishes that is now available, healthy eating is more enjoyable eating

2   Plenty of fruit and vegetables form the basis of healthy eating: vegetarians have better health than meat-eaters and live longer

3   No food is bad for you but red meats,dairy foods, salt and salty foods should be eaten in moderation, and high-fat and starchy foods should be strictly limited in people who are overweight

1   If you smoke cigarettes, giving up is the best and only way to protect your health. Smoking a pipe and cigars are less harmful because such smokers seldom inhale, but these habits are becoming socially unacceptable, lead to poor dental health and, very rarely, result in cancer of the lip and tongue

2   Cigarette smokers have an average lifespan of twenty years less than nonsmokers, and smokers are twice as likely to be off work, ill and in hospital as non-smokers and former smokers

3   Help from various sources is available on giving up smoking: speak to your GP or contact one of the relevant voluntary or government agencies, such as the Irish Heart Foundation, the Irish Cancer Society and the Department of Preventive Medicine at St Vincent's Hospital in Dublin

1   Drink only in moderation, or not at all. Drinking
        in moderation will not harm your health, but
        recent media statements which say that moderate
        drinking improves your health can be taken with
        a grain of salt

2   The recommended weekly limit of alcohol con-
        sumption is twenty-one units for men, fourteen
        for women (a glass of wine, half-pint of beer, or
        measure of spirits is one unit)

3   Make rules about drinking, such as limiting your
        self to a certain number of drinks per week or not
        drinking on certain days of the week

4   Ensure that you are in control of your alcohol con-
        sumption, rather than the other way around

DRUGS

1   All addictive and non-prescribed drugs should be strictly avoided

2   Mild over-the-counter painkillers, such as aspirin or paracetamol, can be taken for odd pains and aches but the instruction on the package must be closely followed. Do not take these painkillers regularly and for long periods without consulting your medical adviser

3   If you are taking a variety of prescribed drugs, particularly over a long period, you should check with your doctor to ascertain the reasons for such prolonged medication, to ensure that the drugs do not conflict by causing side-effects and that they are not having an adverse effect on your health. Avoid being part of the 'drug culture', whether prescribed, over-the-counter or illicit

RISK-TAKING

1   Avoid unnecessary risk of injury at all stages of your life

2   Remember that people who are suffering from stress or are disorganised are more prone to risk

3   Be aware that accidents among old people in the home and on the street, even if trivial, may cause a serious and progressive deterioration in health and quality of life. Such accidents can be prevented with a little care

1   Close family relationships, with links between all generations, create a more stable psychological environment and have been shown to have a pos itive impact on physical health

2   Maintaining close friendships is important, particularly as we get older and retire, when it is easy to become more reclusive

3   Try to have a positive outlook on life. Research has shown that this is one of the best ways of recovering from serious illness and maintaining good health

4   Keep you mind active: read regularly, do a crossword and develop other interests

5   Remember that exercise has benefits for mental health, including helping to alleviate depression

EPILOGUE

As I approached my eightieth birthday I thought it might be appropriate to go on a walking holiday with my wife, Louise, in France. Exercise – tennis, walking, cycling and golf – has been an important component of her life too. We joined a British rambling group for a long week in Burgundy. We spent four days in Vezelay, a small hillside town famous for its great Gothic cathedral, the Basilica of Marie Magdalene, and for its role many centuries ago as one of the starting points of the pilgrimage to Santiago de Compostela in Spain. We spent another four days in Beaune, famous for its wine and its six-hundred-year-old hospice.

France is an ideal country for walking and trekking, as it has a vast network of tracks, paths and laneways. At no time did we walk on the roads or encounter traffic. The countryside here is hilly and ideal for firm walking. It is dotted with numerous woodlands, mostly hardwoods, birch, alder, oak and hazel, with patches of Scots pine and other evergreens. There are many uncut pastures with a wealth of wild flowers, fields of barley and sweetcorn, and a few scattered vineyards. Within the environs of Beaune, about fifty kilometres away, the landscape is almost entirely vineyards as far as the eye can see.

There are few houses scattered around the French countryside. This is in great contrast with the situation in Ireland, where farmhouses are traditionally built on the farm and where in many coastal areas numerous holiday bungalows have been built, with little attention to traditional design and less to proper planning. We are a country of rural as well as suburban sprawl. By contrast, in France, as in many other parts of Europe, the farmers and other country inhabitants live in villages or hamlets. The

155

agricultural areas are clearly well managed and cared for, while the numerous woodlands and areas of scrub, and the natural hedgerows, combined with the absence of dwellings, make for a rich wildlife. Around Strasbourg, where we spent the second week of our holiday, many satellite villages and small towns are linked to the city by excellent roads and cycle pathways. They are a substitute for our suburban sprawl.

We started each morning about ten o'clock. We walked until after midday and, after an hour's rest stretching in the sun, and a picnic, we would walk again until about four in the afternoon. After a stretch of fifteen to eighteen kilometres, we reached base invariably physically tired but mentally exhilarated. The afternoons were warm and sunny, adding a great sense of physical freedom and relaxation among us walkers, who were lightly clad in light shirts or singlets.

A walking holiday is unlike holidays where boredom may make the prospect of returning home more agreeable than going away. A day's walking in the countryside followed by a few hours' rest and relaxation makes for a healthy appetite, enhanced in France by a good *vin du pays*, an excellent night's sleep and, above all, a sense of fulfilment and physical well-being. It also greatly increases one's interest in one's surroundings and is a reminder that we are an integral part of nature and completely dependent on it for our well-being and survival. The visit to France was a fitting event to celebrate my eightieth birthday.

*

I retired from hospital work in 1988. These last fifteen years have been perhaps the most enjoyable of my life. For this I can thank my continuing good health, the support I receive from family and friends, and my many leisure interests.

It is possible to improve with age. With our knowledge of disease and its prevention nowadays, there is no reason why most people cannot live out and enjoy a normal biological lifespan before passing quietly and gently to their reward. The serenity of the elderly, about which we hear so much but see so little, can be achieved by careful planning during our earlier years, by adapting and reconciling ourselves to the physical limitations which are inseparable from our declining years, and by being philosophical about our loss of friends, our removal from the corridors of power and our gradual approach to eternity. This life, with its ups and downs, its joys and sorrows, its triumphs and tragedies, and its inevitable end, is preferable to the meaningless immortality of the gods.

Further Reading and Resources

Aurelius, Marcus. *Meditations.* Penguin Classics, Harmondsworth, 1964.

Cooper, Kenneth H. *Running Without Fear.* M. Evans & Co., New York, 1985.

Dishman, Rod K. *Exercise Adherence: Its Impact on Public Health.* Human Kinetics Books, Champaign, Illinois, 1988.

Fixx, James F. *The Complete Book of Running.* Random House, New York, 1977.

_____. *The Complete Runner's Day-by-day Log and Calendar.* Random House, New York, first published 1971.

Fries, James F. and Lawrence M. Crapo. *Vitality and Ageing: Implications of the Rectangular Curve.* W. H. Freeman and Co., San Francisco, 1981.

Glaver, Bob and Shelly-Lynn Florene. *The Competitive Runner's Handbook.* Penguin Books, Harmondsworth, 1999.

Heathcote, Felicity. *Peak Performance.* Wolfhound Press, Dublin, 1996.

Liston, Dr Richard and Dr Eamon C. Mulkerrin, eds. *Medicine for Older Patients: Cases and Practice.* Health Education Publishers, Dublin, 2003.

Lynam, Joss, ed. *Best Irish Walks.* Gill & Macmillan, Dublin, 2000.

Mulcahy, Risteárd. *Beat Heart Disease.* Martin Dunitz, London, 1979.

_____. *The Long-term Management of Coronary Heart Disease.* Churchill, London, 1989.

Putnam, Robert. *Bowling Alone: The Collapse and Revival of American Community.* Simon & Schuster, New York, 2000.

Rotello, Bob. *Golf is Not a Game of Perfect.* Simon & Schuster, New York, 1995.

Rowland Whitt, Frank and David Gordon Wilson. *Bicycling Science.* The MIT Press, London, 1999.

Chris Sidwells, *The Complete Bike Book.* Dorling & Kindersley, London, 2003.

William Stokes, *Diseases of the Heart and Aorta.* Hodges and Smith, Dublin, 1853

ARTICLES, REPORTS AND WEBSITES

'Muscle, Genes and Athletic Performance'. *Scientific American,* September 2000. www.sciam.com

Interim Report on Exercise and Obesity. Centre for Sports Science and Health. Dublin City University, 2003.

The Lord Mayor's Commission on Cycling. Dublin Corporation, 1995.

Obesity reports include *Obesity in Europe: The Case for Action,* from the International Obesity Task Force, www.iotf.org and *National Nutritional Survey, 2003* and *Obesity Working Report, 2003,* from the Department of Health and Children, Dublin www.doh.ie. Information about organizations that help people control their weight is available at www.weightwatchers.ie and www.unis-lim.ie. Overeaters Anonymous can be contacted on 01-278 8106.

General medical information is available at www.pubmed.ie and information about health in Ireland is available at www.doh.ie. Information about walking, hill-climbing and walking clubs can be obtained from the Mountaineering Council of Ireland, www.mountaineer-ing.ie. For walking holidays outside Ireland, try the Ramblers Association, at www.ramblers.org, or Ramblers' Holidays, at www.ramblersholidays.co.uk.